Alzheimer's Averted

A Path to Survival

Christine Frances Baum VanRyzin

ELEMENTAL BASIC PUBLISHING
APPLETON, WI

Alzheimer's Averted: A Path to Survival
Copyright © 2004 by Christine Frances Baum VanRyzin

Published by Elemental Basic Publishing
P.O. Box 571
Appleton, WI 54912
www.elementalbasicpub.com

Library of Congress Cataloging in Publications Data

VanRyzin, Christine Frances Baum.
Alzheimer's averted : a path to survival / Christine Frances Baum VanRyzin.
—1st ed.—Appleton, WI : Elemental Basic Publishing, 2004
P. ; cm.
Includes bibliographical references and index.
ISBN: 0-9761336-0-1
1. Alzheimer's disease. 2. Alzheimer's disease—Prevention.
3. Alzheimer's disease—Patients—Care.
4. Alzheimer's disease—Patients—Family relationships.
5. Alzheimer's disease—Treatment.   I. Title.

RC523 .V36 2004   2004112742
616.8/31—dc22   0412

Cover Photograph by Wade VanRyzin
Author's and Author's Family Photograph by Ken Cobb Photography

Printed in the U.S.A.
First Edition

Disclaimer

The information presented in this book has been obtained from authentic and reliable sources. Although great care has been taken to ensure the accuracy of the information presented, the author and the publisher cannot assume responsibility for the validity of all the materials or the consequences for their use.

Partnership with your physician, before starting any regimen of vitamins or supplements. The information presented is meant to increase your knowledge and thus further expand your choices.

Dedicated to

Family, Friends and Strangers,

Here and past,

Unaware of which spoken word or act

That has made a difference

In my life

Preface

With the death of our mother came some of the answers to a 20 year mystery. We found she had been suffering from an early onset form of Alzheimer's Disease carrying with it a 50% hereditary factor. Even with the information we gained by her autopsy, this disease does not fit into today's medical knowledge.

I am their third child of nine. Even before our mother's death, it had become apparent that I had inherited some of her genes. Some I am most grateful for, she was a beautiful woman, others impose a challenge. At age 55, I have been journeying for the past 15 years through the same labyrinth that took our mother. Because this disease is so silent, and does not fit into any known description, it has taken years and years to be understood. Being a very "have-to-know" person, I continue to search for the answers, guided with the knowledge from our mother which continues even after her death.

I often do not know the loss until I am facing it, and so I express not so much what I cannot do today, but more about my struggle to relearn. Like chopping an onion. I cannot say "Today I awoke and I no longer know how to chop an onion." Instead, one day I'll have the onion before me with a knife in my hand and I am stuck. I know I was very good at cutting nice, even diced pieces and it is a mystery as to what has happened to that knowledge. In the end my pieces are large and ill-sized. How did I do it before?

An early start has given us time and we have been able to slow the progression, by looking beyond the boundaries.

Fitting the small puzzle pieces together, one by one, we are close to finding its "all". Knowing a cure will be in sight, I have been one of the lucky ones who can still see what is happening and struggle to change it.

When I first began to write, it was for my family. I wanted to be sure they had the information I had found in case one day I was unable to share it. The poems and writings came as a bonus. Perhaps to keep me on track. I share the poems and writings, not because they are exceptionally good, but to show how I had to take an emotion or feeling and once again learn to put it into a thought. How I had to train my brain to once again "find the right word." How I found beauty in life.

Now that I am able to slow the progression I feel a strong responsibility with those whose lives have changed due to Alzheimer's Disease. In reading the articles written on the Internet I am struck by the fact that no one has found the same information. They write of their daily lives and their coping, but it is most often downhill.

As I sort and reread all the books and articles for this book, I learn so much more. I find a strong overlapping among so many diseases: Alzheimer's; stroke; heart; Parkinson's; thyroid; cancer; MS; Diabetes; ALS; Fibromyalgia; and more. So I now want to broaden my reach.

What I have found has not only helped me relearn to live, but may also prove to be the protection our children and grandchildren need to prevent these diseases. Perhaps by sharing, it will help keep one more family intact.

Chris

Milestones

Alzheimer's Averted
A Path to Survival

"Learn to Listen
With
Your Heart"

Chapter I

World War II

The 100 & 18th Evac
With everything strapped on our back
No white sheets or dishes,
But those are our wishes

So cheer up our lads
Love us all

The long, short, the tall
In field shoes and britches
We straddle our ditches

So cheer up our lads
Love us all

Buelah Rose Mancl
1945

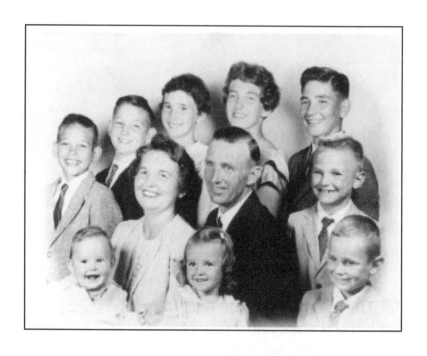

Family Photo
August 1962

Edward, Richard, Christine, Mary Kay, John
Buelah, Vince, Kenneth
Rodger, Rosann, Charles

Our mother was a healer, a nurse, educated when a lot of her peers were unable to financially complete high school. She served during WWII in the army as a nurse. Although her life took on a new meaning when, after the war, she and her new husband accepted the responsibility of his family farm, she never stopped "nursing" and caring for those around her. Their own family grew to include nine children. She instilled in each of us the importance of knowledge and the natural instinct of caring for others. We each have developed this in our own way.

I feel with my whole being that she will never allow any one of her children to suffer with Alzheimer's Disease the way she did. I have felt her with me from the moment of her death when she was free of the devastation that took over her body. She now knows the answers. She now sees the whole picture. It is affecting millions of people in various degrees. She is a nurse, her goal is strong.
Guiding me.

I am now a SURVIVOR. After fifteen years of searching, I continue to seek and find more information that makes each day better instead of worse. I have felt what it was like to have aged to 90. I have faced the beast that took our mother, aunt, and descendants before us whom I have never met. The beast that takes a bit of others every day.

With this healing, comes the responsibility of sharing this information with others. Maybe it will help one family more.

It's been so long since we've heard the sound of her voice.
Hours have turned to days, days to weeks,
weeks to months, and months to years. Do we
even remember the tone?
And yet she is here before us.

Does she even know
who we are? Does she know
where she is - who she is?

There would be the occasional response - a smile
or laugh at her husband's jokes. Did she respond
because she really understood or at
the other sounds of laughter around her?

How is it we are even able to laugh
when such an awful devastation sits before us?
Except, yes, it is what she would have done - it is
what she has taught us each.

She gave us her all every day, every minute
of every day. This unselfish wife, mother,
caregiver of the needy, the moving spirit in
families, neighborhoods, clubs and communities.

It was she who organized the family reunions,
the birthday parties - the celebrations large or small.
It was she who the neighbors called before the doctors.
It was she who reassured the young families.
It was she who taught us to give,
to always be there.

How can you let a spirit like hers go?
How do you ever stop needing her here?
How do you allow the change - to become
the one who needs all the needing
Without losing the dignity she deserves.

LEARN TO LISTEN WITH YOUR HEART!

Her world is mute, this we know
It is worse than mute - it holds
no physical communication. No hands
that can sign, no words that can be written.

How do we hear? The mouth that opens
when food is presented. The slight turn of the head
in no particular direction with the sound of your voice.
The abstract reaching of her arms
at the scent of a spring lilac.

A tear!
What do we feel but panic! Another tear
follows - and another.
How do we fix the unknown!

We were riding down to that great hospital.
The only place to seek help. One of many centers
of teaching, healing, and research. So many trips,
so many years - always going with the same hope.

Maybe this time they will know the answer.
Maybe this time they will find the cure.
This time we will get her back! But how can they cure
what they can't even name?

It was the usual drive. Familiar sights changing
with the seasons and the years. Such slow
changes in this rural drive across the state.
What was new was the car we rode in.

Its biggest feature being a four-door,
not that it would have mattered before,
but it had become a necessity now
As so many other insignificant things had become.

She was still able to walk if you guided her.
Another loss - her freedom to walk
around the house, the yard - at her own free will.
To always now be guided to where
she had no intention of going - and to be left
unable to go where she desired.
How could we know?

So she had been guided to the back seat of the car.
The door was smaller and easier to get in and
propped up with pillows for comfort
she would be more comfortable. We could
attend to her easier if she rode there.
From the front seat I could reach back
and give her a drink - make sure she was OK.
Husband and daughter sat in the front seat
commenting on the changes in the outside world.

"Yes, the geese were making their annual trip south.
Yes, the farmers' fields were dry for harvest.
Yes, the road construction ..."
Oh, the tears... Many tears rolling down her face!
Questions, questions !

Check is she too warm... is she slumping over...
she refuses a drink! Think! Find an answer.
Reassure her as to where she is,
where we are going. Maybe she needs a stop.

OK - reassure her we will stop, as soon as
we reach the next town. The tears continue
to roll down her soft check. How much further?
There - next exit - a fast food restaurant. Pull in.
Yes, daughter take her in - guide her slowly.

The struggle of it all - the loss of another piece of dignity
to be unable to perform this natural act unattended
Now timed each day by the hour and not by the need.
Like a child in training.

Another loss, another display of humility.
How humble before mankind must she become
before she is released from this devastation.
Lest we know...
It had only just begun!

On the slow walk back, I seek
my father's questioning eyes – was this stop
the answer? A shake of my head to indicate
no. She felt no need, the tears are still there.
Our hearts break a little more.

What? What? 'Learn to feel with your heart.'
'Learn to listen with your Heart.'
'Learn to Listen with your Heart!'
I glance at that new car - so shiny...

'Learn to LISTEN with your HEART!' That's IT!
"She wants to sit in the front!" I proclaim!
Father looks at daughter questioning.
"Her place is in the front seat, next to you, as always."

Tears roll down his stressed checks.
How can he learn to hear?
How can he watch this devastation?
What does he need to do - to give - to stop this?
When will his wife return?
Where will the strength come from?

From their love – it is what she taught us!
She is settled into the front seat. Yes, if we tilt
the seat back a bit and put the arm rest down,
I can reach her from the back seat. It will be
a bit of a struggle, but it can be done.

The drive continues on and she turns her head
in no particular way as the comments about
the changing world are heard.
The tears have stopped. She drifts off into a restful sleep.

She is and always will be the wife and mother.
A lesson learned that day
To never be challenged again.

LEARN TO LISTEN WITH YOUR HEART!

Let Me Be Me

Hold onto the Me inside
Hidden away in changes of age seen too soon

I long to stay free enough to laugh and cry
But the smiles that were once so soft
                    come now with stiffness

Inside there should be screams of injustice
But there is only a growing void

Do not let it take the Me

Remember Me
I was once the tender touch upon
                    your shoulder ... The Supporter
I was once the gentle squeeze of
                    your hand ... The Comforter

Lift the void that surrounds Me
Come touch me with Love
            for then ...
                    I am still Me

Her name is Buelah Rose - Buelah
spelled with the u before the e. That makes
the difference. She was named after a favorite Aunt
of her mother's. But that was still a heavy name to bear.

She did well in those earlier years to hide
the changes she felt. Her afternoon naps
no concern, she was up early. The Sunday chicken,
Monday wash and roast beef, Tuesday ironing and
hamburger, etc. It was seen as a routine,
actually a comfort.

As they started traveling, there were
separate sets of clothes - always washed,
ironed, and folded, placed into plastic bags
in a certain drawer. She was so proud of that one.

Not until later did I see the need and
was amazed at her resourcefulness.
Being an at-home housewife with a capital H,
she was able to function without detection.

Not until the phone calls came.
She wasn't sure why she was calling me,
she just had to talk for a bit...
        Isolation

We'd talk, sometimes for an hour or more.
Most times I'd pack up my little ones
into our red wagon and walk out to spend the day,
feigning the need for garden tomatoes
or advice on a recipe.

The grandchildren made her happy
but they, too, sensed a change and
always played quietly or drew pictures.
      Isolation

She separated from the clubs and committees
that were such an important part of her life.
She was a leader. She had been instrumental
in setting up a county health-care system. One by
one she dropped from the clubs and organizations.
Until there were no meetings to attend.
      Isolation

The family saw – "We need to get help for you!"
"No, No" The tears ran down her face.
'If my family sees it, then it must be real
 this awful thing cannot be real!'
Her husband speaks, "Listen to your daughters,
they are trying to tell you something".

The secret is out. 'No this cannot be real
why it was just a few years back that I
was nursing your mother, she was troubled
and often confused, but she was 80
I'm only 56. Too young to lose my identity.'
        Isolation

This is a disease filled with mystery. It takes
on many faces. Affecting each a little different,
depending upon the damage that is being done.
If a great murder mystery of the 90's were to be written
this would be a good case!

Is it all in the genes? And how come it seems
so hard to find evidence in the past generations?
It was not to be talked about. Certainly not to be
recorded. "Died from brain impairment"
Wow - "witches" were burnt at the stake for less!

And then why don't all or 50% have it
like the figures say. But then half her family died
young - in their early 60's or younger.
Most from heart problems so maybe we weren't aware.
        Isolation

WE ARE HERE

IT STARTS SO QUIETLY - NO ONE KNOWS - I KNOW
THE WALLS GO UP - THEY ARE SO CLEAR -
   BUT THERE

I SENSE THEM BEFORE I FEEL THEM
   WHAT HAS HAPPENED?

SMILE AT ME - I SEE YOU THROUGH A WINDOW
TOUCH ME - I CAN FIND THE DOOR
HUG ME - I AM BACK WITH YOU

Buelah Rose died September 16, 1995.
Even those last years when she could not do
one thing for herself - she still gave. Her caretakers
would comment on what a loving person she was.

How could they know? What was left of her to share?
It was her Heart!
LEARN TO LISTEN WITH YOUR HEART!
This magnificent lady - wife, mother, sister, friend
Was still teaching to the end.

I am their third child of nine. Even before her death
it had become apparent that I had inherited some of her
genes. Some I am most grateful for, she was a beautiful
woman. Others impose a challenge.

"When one door closes - another will open."
I was terrified - there was no way I wanted to be looking
down the throat of this beast that brings so much pain
and separation. The idea of losing who I am,
the change in going from being depended upon to
being a dependent is very hard on a family.

I have not been alone. Family and friends,
here and past, pull me back each time I take that
misstep, unaware of which spoken word or act that
has made a difference in my life.
To each one I belong.

"Laughter is the best medicine"
my husband's golden rule surrounded
by love. Not giving up if he receives
barely a formed smile. Knowingly he will
pump up those endorphins
until laughter comes with tears.

His wisdom and insight is unending.
With nights and nights of eluded sleep
due to an uncontrolled brain running like
a lost train... faster and faster, he simply states

"Maybe you should write it down."
How can that help? But it did. Writing and writing
until exhausted - sleep finds me.

Encouraged by a daughter who gave me
empty journals to fill; who gave me
my dignity; who left me my worth.
And listened to by a son who shares
my imaginary world full of creativity - but there,
beside me, to keep one foot in reality.

I have found some hidden parts of me. In having
to slow down I have been able to
Listen with my heart!

It has been good to explore
what else I am made of. Every minute
of every day is now important to me and
is shared with my family and friends.
A lot of people don't get to feel that.

And so, I take this time to share with you
"my voice from my heart" - like my mother did
for all those years of "silence."

Maybe this is what we
should be doing all along...

Aging

Young – Old
Life – Death
One can age and feel so young
Be old and feel so full of life
When has death taken over life?
When you feel old and death
Takes who you are -
Be it fast or slow.
When am I more dead than alive?
Age – the years can be counted
Death – how can it be measured,
"One foot in the grave" ?

As the devastation continued throughout our mother's body, we always hoped that she never "felt" or "knew" what was happening.

How could she not -
It was the only thing left of Her -
Feelings

August 1989

I am the matron-of-honor at our younger sister's wedding. The
flowers I carry are of a very "artsy" style with long, twisty tubules
extending from the bouquet. Greeting people in the receiving line
after the ceremony, numerous relatives ask if I am OK. They relate
that my bouquet never stopped shaking. (Other people are now
seeing what I have been feeling... the tremors.) Later as I review
the photographs, I break down and cry... I do not look like I used to.
My face is very stiff and "frozen" looking. My sister suggests I talk
with a doctor.

My mother and I have the same family doctor. I chose her because
she would understand what we as a family are going through. So
when I come to her with my fears; the symptoms of failing memory,
feeling less intelligent, and tremors, over the past two years; she is
very quick to send me down to the University to see the specialists
who are treating our mother.

My appointment is at the University of Wisconsin Hospital Clinic with
Dr. Benjamin Brooks, neurology. He patiently takes down a family
and health history (including all jobs, travel, environmental issues,
and accidents). This diagnosis, like our mother's, can only be made
by the *process of eliminating* all other diseases. And then only a
"probable" statement can be made.

The testing is very extensive. Extensive blood work, MRI of the
brain, EEG, and neuropsychological testing are but a few of the
tests. I am familiar with all of them, as our mother has also been
through these tests.

Before I am able to return for the answers, I have a morning of extreme vertigo. Even with my eyes closed the room is spinning around me. I call my husband home from work and he takes me into our family doctor. After a check-up I am sent back home. The vertigo lasts for 5 hours. For days after I have "fumbling fingers" and my walking is "off." In the years to come we will learn that this vertigo is one of the "un-silent" clues that damage is being done. What type of damage will remain a mystery for many more years.

In returning to the University I am told that the only positive results are from the neuropsychological exam for depression. Well, that rules out a lot of the "simple things." I expected answers. But why? At this point they still have no idea what is causing our mother's decline. They hadn't seen her until she was already incapacitated and do not know the early problems. But we as a family do.

Silence... silently, it steals parts of you, most often leaving no trail or only a trail hidden deep. By the time it is visible, the damage is so great. I don't want to wait until then.

So I am "documented," a baseline. Told to keep a very good diary. Come back if things change. The diary becomes the basis of this book.

The frustrations of going to a medical facility - each time with new hope. The car ride back, searching through the information received that day, hoping someone else heard something that you missed.

Trying to understand just what was and wasn't said.
Trusting that the answer will come... Perhaps next time.

It's ironic - "They," the medical profession, say, "Early
diagnosis is your only chance." And yet they (the
neuropsychologists) appear to be doing everything to
disclaim you. "Yes, you have some cognitive decline - but
it's probably due to the fact that you are depressed."
Wow - which came first, the chicken or the egg?

How can you join a support group or get anyone to talk to?
"Hi, my name is Chris. I don't know if I belong here, they
can't tell me until I die. And although I look fine to you,
inside a piece of me is lost every day. But it is OK if you see
me as a stranger - because I feel like a stranger to myself."
                    And hey, that's Isolation

My greatest fear when seeing a doctor or therapist:
        "You don't believe me or believe in me."
Because I can't fix this and if you don't believe in me - you
who have access to the knowledge - I have no chance at all.
                        Isolation

How do I act?
  1) Ignore the symptoms
  2) Keep pushing, ignoring the warnings
  3) Accept
  4) Fight
  5) Research - Seek
  6) Plan

7) Pretend
8) Act - Role play
9) Faith
10) Depend on others

I choose   *Research - Seek*

It's like starting a new job or a new class in school. You start at the edge looking in, wondering if you will come to the point of being comfortable with all the strange information that sits before you.
I'm on a path.
Medicine, the body, the BRAIN.
How am I to ever understand its workings,
the complexity of it all,
the mystery?

I remember taking a yoga class years back. After several lessons I found I was hearing my heart beat at different times throughout the day. If I could learn to connect with my heartbeat, then I can just as easily learn to connect with my brain and find the answers to this mystery disease.

This world of ours... you can feel it getting smaller and smaller. Where trust in the human race as a whole has to be achieved. We depend on countries, companies, other human beings of all backgrounds for our health, food, and our very existence. Our lives are in each others' hands.
So as East meets West, I look beyond boundaries for answers.

Winter 1990
As I sit in my car outside the bank, with the sun shining to
warm the crisp winter air, I experience my first feeling of
"not being sick!" It doesn't last long, fleeting by, but real all
the same.

What had I done? How can I repeat this? Is there hope?
A smile teases at my cheeks.

And then I'm tugged back to feeling like 90 years old when I
had only celebrated 42.

The next day another passing feeling of "not being sick."
This time a bit longer. Can there really be hope?
By the third day, I am sure it is not my imagination.
The vitamins I had started the previous days are making a
difference.

And the road back begins. And with it, the start of the
research to find the answers...
often viewed as an obsession.
Where to begin?

I start my quest for knowledge at the public library researching articles held in the vertical files as I find there are but a
few books written to help. It is there that I realize the
information on Alzheimer's Disease and related Parkinson's
Disease is very limited. Without a firm diagnosis, I add in all
neurological diseases, finding that most of them overlap.

The experience with our mother gives us almost an equal amount of information. And so I start my own collection of books and references. Maybe if I document it, someone, later down the line, will find my notes and know the answer. The first book, of many, I have read to find the information to better understand what is happening.

The Amazing Brain   1984
   Robert Ornstein & Richard F. Thompson
   Illustrated by David Macaulay
   Houghton Mifflin Company, Publisher
Starting with the basics, I find a book that explains the parts of the brain and how they work. So much more has been discovered since my high school biology classes — most of it starting in the 1980's. This has been a little too late for our mother, but we have future generations to help.

Our mother, being a nurse, had always kept a special, thick, well-worn book handy. It was *Taber's Cyclopedic Medical Dictionary*. As kids we used to sneak it off the high shelf and sit ever so quietly (if you can imagine that) and page carefully through it. So when I saw the latest edition (#17) sitting on the bookstore shelf, I knew I needed to purchase it. It does not hold the beautifully colored illustration plates our mother's copy did, but the information will prove to be just as important. (Perhaps this is step one of her guidance.)

There are numerous books that are based on the Eastern philosophy of healing. Each instructing you in the basic "what" to do. And up until now, I have not found a book on the "why". *Quantum Healing* by Deepak Chopra, M.D. (Bantam Books, 1990) addresses this scientific approach to Eastern medicine, which my analytical mind needs. He takes away the "leap in faith" basis and presents the powerful healing ability of the mind and body in a very easy to understand format.

I must admit that in rereading the book after all these years, I did not remember many of the actual facts from when I first read it. I do, however, find that I have used this information, without realizing it, as a strong basis for my healing. You may recognize this throughout my writing.

> *Quantum Healing* by Deepak Chopra, copyright © 1989 by Deepak Chopra, M.D. Used by permission of Bantam Books, A division of Random House, Inc *Exploring the Frontiers of Mind/Body Medicine*
>
> A level of total, deep relaxation is the most important precondition for curing any disorder. The body knows how to maintain balance unless thrown off by disease.
>
> Just before the cure appears, almost every patient experiences a dramatic shift in awareness. He knows that he will be healed, and he feels that the force responsible is

inside himself but not limited to him - it extends beyond his personal boundaries, throughout all of nature. The word that comes to mind when a scientist thinks of such sudden changes is *quantum*. The word denotes a discrete jump from one level of functioning to a higher level - the quantum leap. The healing process includes getting well in mind and body at the same time. The mind-body system knows that the process of healing is under way and may begin to generate positive thoughts simultaneously.

Intelligence is present everywhere in our bodies. It directs the actual matter of the body. If you could see your body as it really is, you would never see it the same way twice. Ninety-eight percent of the atoms in your body were not there a year ago. The skeleton that seems so solid was not there three months ago. The skin is new every month.

Just before falling asleep, the mind gradually leaves the waking state, withdrawing the senses, shutting out the waking world. At the junction point before the mind actually falls asleep, a brief gap is opened, identical to the one that flashes by between each thought. It is silence. When the brain is thinking, it is all activity; when it stops thinking, it returns to its source in silence. Meditation, accesses silence and leads the mind to a "free zone" that is not touched by disease. Afterward, when the mind returns to its usual level of consciousness it has acquired a little freedom to move, thus allowing the body to get unstuck from the disease.

Together, meditation, bliss, and primordial sound are the tools of quantum healing. All three participants share equally in what gets said - what the mind knows is also known by the body and DNA.

Bliss is when reality takes on splendor; experiencing grandeur and peace, mighty and majestic, or power and beauty. Bliss is a continuous signal that connects mind, body, and DNA.

The vibrational sound called Om is used as a specific signal to repair the break. It's like reminding the body of what station it should be tuned. It is no accident that the syllable Om sounds like the English "hum". When Eastern rishis tuned into the sound of the universe, they actually heard it as a cosmic hum.

Quantum healing is the ability of the mind to spontaneously correct the mistakes in the body.

Thoughts...
The biggest news to us is the new realization that the brain is repairable and holds the intelligence to repair. Up to now, and throughout our mother's disease, it was believed that any damage done would be permanent. Doctors and researchers felt the only chance was prevention, slowing the destruction, or stopping it completely. None of which they are able to do. You would always be left where you were with the damage done. So now we are given "hope." Although no one can tell us how this will happen... but maybe tomorrow.

Quantum Healing has given me some good "mind set" images. The thought of new cells replacing other cells and making new body parts on a continuous basis is most reassuring. I remember talking about skin cells in biology but I never put it to the whole body. So why can't I reprogram the cells that have gone astray? First I have to know where they are and exactly what is wrong with me. We still don't know. Chanting is something I have had a hard time with. I had put it on the "back burner" for a while. But referencing it to "humming" is more *Western.* I remember my mother often humming as she worked about the house. It may be a lost art. I also remember the beautiful Latin Gregorian chant that was saved for special occasions in church - all mysterious, and comforting. Perhaps the church should not have been so quick to change it.

I love the word *bliss.* It, by itself, conjures up images of happiness, freedom, and wellness. I try every day to feel the bliss and let the world take care of itself.

One of the earliest books I read that gave me my first introduction into an alternative choice in thinking was

   Jonathan Livingston Seagull by Richard Bach, ©1970

It keeps popping back up as I try to put new meaning to my life. I actually clung to that new perspective. I loved the idea of levels of learning, levels of life. Perhaps it was because of the Vietnam war. The uncertainty of how our lives were going to turn out. The separation of our new small family and the need for new hope. Already in my 20's, I felt life was too short to only experience it once.

Perhaps there was more to life than our set "Western" ideas. That there has to be a higher purpose than just "going to heaven." A little spark set deep in my subconscious for another time. Not knowing then, how important that idea was to become (in just a few short years) when we would be thrown into another personal war, another separation.

How strong my husband is. This road will not be a mystery to him. He sees every step our mother takes.

He knows... He brings me the gift of endorphins. Whether from his endless humor or intimate loving, he makes sure the healing endorphins are circulating throughout my body.

Our mother continues to slip away, ever so slowly...

I remember years ago, my husband's family machine shop was asked to manufacture an important piece for a proto-type diagnostic machine at the University Hospital. The same machine that our mother was lucky enough to be one of the first patients to use. An MRI. It told us a bit of what changes were occurring in the brain, but not the why. I am proud of my husband. We are all trying together to find the answers.

Change in health...
We noted with our mother that her decline was on a stair step rather than a slide. She would have a big loss and gradually work her way back, sometimes almost getting all back, and then she'd have another decline. Until she could no longer get enough back and the declines became larger. I am similar. So in my early stages it is most difficult to find what is wrong. I know what I feel and what I have lost, but the doctors cannot measure it. I am documented again, and told to come back if the "symptoms" persist.

There is a feeling that overwhelms me. I'll be doing my job, and this feeling will start from my toes, flood up my body, disconnecting every part! Watch out for anyone around me because suddenly I cannot cope - I could have been laugh-ing and everything is fine. A question is asked of me and suddenly I blow apart - almost collapsing, I escape the room. As I recognize the beginnings of these feelings, I run to my bedroom or car where I scream at the top of my voice, and then cry...
because I don't understand...

The softness in my face is being replaced by a frightening tight mask. My children are afraid of me. This is not ME. So many ups and downs. Will I be able to slow the "downs" enough to beat this?

I am at a point in my life where my brain won't shut down at night. During the day when I am physically active, my brain does not seem to work. It is like I only have enough energy to do one thing at a time. So during the day, I am walking, talking, eating, etc. and there is not enough energy left to think. At night my body is resting and all the thoughts and memories of the day come rolling out. It feels like a race of thoughts, each one wanting its chance. It's very "unrestfull."

At a physical examination in 1993, it is noted that my blood pressure is elevated. It is suggested that perhaps there have been spikes in my blood pressure that should be controlled. I am given Captopril to take.

That night a very exciting thing happens. In my "unrest," memories of my childhood on the farm roll out. These are the first of memories - memories I felt were forever lost... They were not gone, just unreachable! What a realization! These memories/feelings become the basis for my personal bliss/energy. It is "where I go" to heal. It is where I find the energy flowing from the universe to me.
I write them down in case I "lose" them again......
    CHILDREN OF THE FARM

    See Appendix for full poem.

CHILDREN OF THE FARM

ENDLESS ADVENTURE - BEGINNING

It was an adventurous time
for young children born to the farm
Free to explore and
run with their imaginations.
Fifty years ago when all felt safer.

Born into the best of two worlds
as this farm was set at the edge of a city.
The "edge" was where the bus route was,
So as the children grew
the city awaited only a ride away.

An endless fantasy land
the farm held all the mysteries of
Life past with a promise of the future.

Its energies brought with those
Who had been there before –
waiting to be discovered and cherished…
Held and passed onto those that follow…

Children of the Farm

1995 September
It's the middle of the night. The house
once more holds a vigil of death.
Rooms are filled with family
catching moments of rest
between shifts to nurse and comfort.

Spirits abound opening a bridge
to the past while forming a path
to the future. They take her hand
to show her the way. No longer
inhibited by her body she escapes
that which has held her
imprisoned.

It takes a long time to die. And
during this time if we listen
we will learn...

Our mother is 75 years old when she dies early on September 16, 1995. It has been over 25 years of questioning: "What is happening to me?"

Mama's death is not easy, her passing takes 14 days and nights. During this time, her spirit is free to visit those whom she was unable to speak to for so many long years...

We have made her a "bedroom" in what we called the far living room of the old farmhouse. When I was a child and our grandparents lived here, huge velvet drapes adorned the wooden colonnades between this room and the central living room. This has been Mama's "room" for the past six years. When an adjustable bed and lift were added for her homecare she had to leave her husband's side in the bedroom she had decorated not that long ago. The family had moved from our "little house" to the larger farm house after our grandparents passed away. Mama and I had picked out the wallpaper for their bedroom. She choosing a light pattern of flowers and butterflies. "They will be nice to look at if I have to spend a lot of time in bed."
Did she know?

Narration by my older sister, Mary Kay:
> About 3 or 4 days before Mom actually died, I was at her bedside in the "front room." I was playing tapes and reading Bible psalms. It was late afternoon and no one else was able to be at the homestead at that time.

I heard a woman's voice coming from the kitchen or back door. The voice sounded like one of my Aunts (Mom's sisters) calling out my name. I called back, "Come on in" not really wanting to leave Mom's side. I heard the voice again, saying my name again. I got up and walked to the kitchen, checking the back porch. There was no one there... and no one in the yard either... no cars other than mine. I felt this over- whelming sense of the presence of Mom, however, while still in the kitchen. And I was so overwhelmed with the sense that Mom was still calling me by name - even though I had not heard her say my name for several years. I felt infinitely loved and loveable. The next day we had a very hard time giving Mom pain medicine - she had not swallowed for days. And even though her body twitched and her face scrunched in the appearance of pain, I was calm. I knew Mom was no longer constrained by her body. She was calling to all of us in other ways.

Our younger sister, Rosann, related later that she, too, had heard Mama call her name even though she has not had the ability to speak for years. While in the kitchen, Rosann clearly heard her name called out from the front living room. Hurrying in to answer, she finds her sleeping peacefully.

And so, I too...

As I walk outside, I feel her become a part of me. I can feel her about and in me like thick pudding. Using my body to feel, see and hear she leads me through her gardens, reaching out to touch the rough bark of the trees, feel the grass under foot, and smell the air scented with fall, one more time. I can feel her spirit free - knowing her ravaged body and pain are left behind. Tears roll down my check even as a smile crosses my mouth. There is a feeling of sadness for our separation, yet joy for her transformation. "Who she is" is now whole.

She is showing us how we are to feel her presence. We know, now, that she will always be there for us.

We are truly allowed to see and experience a new level of life.

A Parent Sees... is written with my pencil on the paper before me, sitting at her dining room table the day of her death. The words flow onto the paper with hardly a thought - they are her words...
She writes... She leads me...

They are read at her funeral.

A Parent Sees...

My Child
Do not Fear or Weep for the
 Times Spent apart

Know that You need not be Close
 To share your Life with Me
 For I See what You See...
 I Feel what You Feel

Thru You I experience Worlds
 Unattainable to Me
 For I am of You

Look with Respect onto this World
 Bringing with it Love

Spread your Wings
 Go near or far...
 So that I too may Fly
  With You
  Thru You
  Forever...

We learn the "what." With the autopsy report we have our answers to the "what," but not the "why or how" of our mother's disease. We also face the truth that as her heirs there is a 50% hereditary factor, which was suspected when her younger sister was also afflicted.

Autopsy:

Her posterior dementia was due to a combination of Alzheimer's Disease with amyloid angiopathy. Alzheimer's Disease is characterized by changes that we can define specifically on the microscopic examination by the presence of a large number of plaques and neurofibrillary tangles. In addition, she had Granulovacuolar degeneration and PAS plaques. The amyloid angiopathy is a particular familial form of Alzheimer's disease. The unique feature was the presence of lacunar changes (e'tat lacunaire) in the basal ganglia and cribriform changes in the cerebral white matter (e'tat cribre'). The patient also had evidence of involvement of the substantia nigra, locus caeruleus, but no significant abnormality in the left meninges. This neuro degeneration brings together under the diagnostic heading Alzheimer's Disease with amyloid angiopathy the realization that this is probably a familial disease. At the present time, there is no specific DNA test that would identify who in the future may have this condition. Much research is being carried forward in trying to identify people who may have this condition with a genetic test so that early prophylactic treatment can be instituted. At the present time, we have no such treatment and the attempts to develop this treatment are under way at several major universities.

What will this all mean to us?
We now know the "What" - but we do not know the "How" and
the "Why." I have an empty, sinking, feeling in my chest.
Will we be able to find enough information to stop this in just
a few years... it is all I have.

Some hope is found in the book, *Brain Repair*
authored by: Donald G. Stein, Professor of Psychobiology and
Vice-Provost and Dean of the Graduate School of Emory
University, Atlanta, Georgia; Simon Brailowsky Professor of
Neuroscience at the National University of Mexico; and Bruno
Will Professor of Neurophysiology and Biology at Louis
Pasteur University, Strasbourg, France.
Oxford University Press, 198 Madison Ave, New York, NY.
Printed with permission.

Giving an insight into how the brain can be injured by
accident or disease, this book takes us through the steps of
brain injury and some new ideas on how repair will take
place. I am overwhelmed with the depth of the information.
But like all the other books, I flag and tag and mark and
make notes.

Will this "How" fit into our "How"?

It is not until seven years later that I am able to fit this
important information into the big puzzle.

Brain Repair   Donald G Stein, Simon Brailowsky and
Bruno Will, 1995©   Oxford University Press
Printed with permission.

Introduction Imagine what it would be like to wake up
one morning and not be able to read this sentence, or to
remember your name, or to hold a cup of coffee. Try to
imagine looking at a familiar object and not being able to
know what it is, or to know exactly what it is, but not be
able to speak its name. *Brain Repair* is written to show
that more can and should be done to help patients
suffering from injury or degenerative disease of the brain.
The results of current, clinical and experimental research
are beginning to change traditionally held ideas about the
brain and how it works.

Chapter 1 Brain and Behavior: A Brief History of Ideas
Knowledge of the brain dates back to the great Pharaohs
of Egypt (about 3500 B.C.). A papyrus taken from a tomb
carefully describes a head injury and gives a fairly
accurate diagnosis of its causes and symptoms.

Chapter 2 Looking into the Living Brain
With the aid of sophisticated computers, tremendous
amounts of information can be processed to create
pictures of the brain with stunning definition, sometimes
in three dimensions, that take on the appearance of a
hologram.

Technologies used are: Fixed X-ray, absorption tomography, CAT scans, PET scans, MRI, and EEG's. Variations of each of these can provide an important role in diagnosis, precision in surgical steps, and give a basis for understanding brain metabolism and chemistry.

Chapter 3 Neurons at Work

There are basically two types of signals that the nerve cells use to conduct information from one place to another in the brain and throughout the body: electrical and chemical (*neurotransmitters*). From these two kinds of signals flow all of our awareness, our intellect, our creativity, our abilities to love or hate, and to procreate.

Chapter 4 The Injured Brain

One of the first changes after a brain trauma occurs is in what is called the *blood-brain barrier*. In a healthy individual, the blood-brain barrier protects the brain from potentially harmful substances that may circulate in the blood. When the blood-brain barrier is disrupted by injury, blood cells, proteins, and other toxic substances can pour into the cellular spaces containing neurons and glia. The extra and unwanted fluids build up rapidly and cause swelling, which is called *edema*.

Glial cells act as sponges and scavengers of the toxic by-products caused by the injury, but when they become over-loaded, they can die and then re-release the toxic chemicals back into cerebral circulation, where they kill additional neurons.

In the earliest phase of the lesion, the injured, dying, and traumatized cells are in a state of shock and release all of their stores of amino-acid neurotransmitters (glutamate and aspartate, etc.) and the calcium ions needed to activate them. The extremely high levels of these substances are sufficient to kill vulnerable and weakened neurons by damaging their membranes or by exciting them to a point where they "burn out" and die.

Over-stimulated excitatory neurons release glutamate into the brain. This excess glutamate introduces a massive amount of calcium into the nerve cells, activating enzymes that kill the neuron from within. This is called *excitotoxicity*. Some neurons located in the immediate area of the trauma do not die right away, but begin to degenerate during the first 24 hours, or weeks or months later.

Blood-borne and injury-produced charged particles of oxygen and iron, called *free radicals*, are also highly toxic to injured neurons.

Chapter 5 Regeneration, Repair, and Reorganization

Different kinds of growth and regeneration can take place in the damaged brain. The big problem to be solved is whether or not the growth has beneficial or detrimental effects, and whether the new growth is needed to sustain the recovery once it has actually occurred.

Chapter 6 Factors in the Brain That Enhance
                Growth and Repair

At the beginning of this century, Ramon y Cajal knew that one possible reason he did not see regeneration in the damaged nervous system could be that the adult brain did not produce enough of the so-called *growth factors* (biochemical compounds) that might help combat the injury and sustain survival. Modern neurobiologists have identified proteins that stimulate growth and guide regenerating neurons to their targets; these are called *neurotrophic factors* (nerve growth factors - NGF). One of the hypotheses about Alzheimer's Disease is that its victims have lost their capacity to make NGF and have begun to lose the cells that produce the neurotransmitter acetylcholine which is implicated in memory formation and storage. One of the most exciting findings in recovery research in recent years is that the injured brain makes its own neurotrophic "healing" factors that can reduce additional neuronal loss.

Glial cells, which are nonneuronal cells, in the brain make, stockpile, and release trophic factors during the course of normal development and in response to injury and disease. Like so many other things in life, it is a question of balance, of proportion, and of timing. Proper balance applies to other systems in the brain as well. We know that some amino acids (which are the building blocks of life) can act like neurotransmitters to excite or inhibit nerve cells. The amino acid glutamate acts as an excitatory transmitter, but when too much is released by over-excited cells, it becomes highly toxic and will begin to kill everything around it.

Chapter 7 Age and Recovery:
Is There a Difference Between Brain Damage That Occurs Early and Late in Life? The type of injury will be the determining factor for the difference in recovery from young to old. While young patients usually recover from aphasia (loss of language ability) sometimes in just a few weeks where it may take years or longer, if ever, in adults; lesions caused by excessive amounts of excitatory amino acids such as glutamate are usually much more severe in the immature brain than in the adult brain. "Momentum of the lesion effect" is a more critical factor, a slow progressing disease as compared to an accident. First, a brain injury is a trauma that may be more disruptive with depression and shock altering the levels

of neurotransmitters, hormones, and toxic substances. Second, the brain's own growth factors are in limited supply, a slower progression will give time for re-supply. Third, there is a reorganization of function as well as structure, including sprouting and regeneration, slowing the effects of the disease. And fourth, brain damaged individuals immediately have to deal with their change and still have to find ways to cope and survive. The less the trauma and crisis (in the brain), the less the alterations in their relationship to the world, and the easier the adaptation.

Chapter 8 Brain Transplants as Therapy for Brain Injuries?

A chapter on the history and new techniques in brain cell/tissue transplants.

Chapter 9 The Pharmacology of Brain Injury Repair

Problems faced in developing wide spread drugs to treat head injury include, first, the nature of the drug. The drug has to be absorbed into membranes, whether in the stomach, liver or blood vessels. It has to be able to cross the blood-brain barrier and then work appropriately in the brain. Second, the patient's own history and health status prior to the injury must be considered, including male or female. Along with the environment of the patient after the injury.

In a recent review, J.T. Dickerson of the University of Surey in England reported that, in normal people, protein contributes about 10 to 15 percent of the energy required for normal body metabolism. In head-injured patients, 160 to 240 percent increases in protein administration were needed to obtain the same level of systemic metabolic activity, where nitrogen was used as the measure of balance. If the metabolic needs of brain-injured patients are not taken into consideration in planning acute and chronic therapy, malnutrition and failure to respond properly to drug therapy could be the outcome. Dickerson also pointed out that muscle wasting and muscle weakness, which often accompany severe head injury, can result from insulin deficiency and over-production of glucose, which in turn can lead to more nerve cell toxicity. Many drugs, especially trophic factors, may be affected by high levels of insulin, or themselves may alter glucose metabolism in ways that might extend or inhibit their effects in the brain. The free-radical peroxidation reactions can be blocked or reduced in the damaged areas with scavengers called *antioxidants*. Vitamin E is one such antioxidant. Substances from Ginkgo Biloba are a virtual pharmacological "cocktail" seemingly prepared by nature precisely to counteract the cascade of events implicated in brain injury. The old reliable analgesic and anti-inflammatory aspirin may be proven helpful.

Chapter 10   Environment, Brain Function and Brain Repair

The new field of "psychoneuroimmunology" is just beginning to address the complexities of how psychological events can influence physiological phenomena in health and disease - including even the mechanism of neuronal repair in response to injury. The problem that we need to solve is how cognitive processes can impact physiology and, in turn, alter the body's response to injury and healing. We also need to overcome the bias in medical research that implicitly assumes that only physical or mechanistic approaches to treatment will be effective - that is, that only surgery, medication, or elimination of a pathogen can heal an organism. We are not saying that the traditional approaches should not be employed when they are appropriate. But as we learn more about contextual or "personal" variables in healing and recovery, we should be willing to explore how they might enhance accepted medical practice, especially since traditional medical practice currently has little to offer in promoting functional recovery from brain or spinal cord injury. Intention and attitude of the patient can play a significant role in influencing therapeutic outcome. The more meaningful the task or intentions, the better the patient's performance in rehabilitation training.

Epilogue   Where Do We Go from Here?

Neural plasticity - the technical term for the ability of the brain to change and repair itself. It may be the case that deficits often do not appear until decades after the initial damage. We need a combination of pharmacological, behavioral, and environmental therapies - the "keys" to unlock and promote the brain's inherent ability to heal itself. What are the critical lessons we have learned from all of this research? First, brain injury must be treated as soon as possible. Second, for the best outcome, both pharmacological and behavioral interventions are needed. Third, careful attention has to be paid to the individual's past history, health status, age, and experience in developing appropriate treatment strategies. Fourth, sensory and cognitive stimulation has to be combined with drug therapy to produce the best results. Enriched and supportive environments may lead to more rapid and long-lasting functional recovery than deprived or uncaring ones. Fifth, duration of treatment cannot be predicted without considering individual differences among patients. Recovery takes far longer than would be expected. Sixth, gender and hormonal status may be important. Lastly, we have seen how attitudes, beliefs, and ideas about the central nervous system have hampered research in the area of recovery. Since the brain takes time to heal, we must give the brain-injured patient that opportunity for healing.

Thoughts...

What are the important facts here?

Brain Repair introduces me to a lot of new terms:

> Blood-brain barrier
>
> Excitotoxins - glutamate and aspartate
>
> Excitotoxicity
>
> Free radicals
>
> Nerve growth factors
>
> Antioxidants
>
> Ginkgo Biloba
>
> Neural plasticity
>
> Cascade of events
>
> Combination of therapies for healing
>
> Protein needs to increase 160 to 240%

Will these fit into our disease?

A Step Back...1995 Health changes...
After the stabilization of the blood pressure and a good winter, the spring of 1995 again brings changes. I have several episodes of dizziness. And May brings tremors in my hands, dropping things easily, and slurring of words. By summer, I can feel the slide backwards. I have stopped "feeling better." My body from the waist down doesn't work right.

I am feeling apart from everyone, and I don't think I'll have energy for the upcoming fall. My daughter suggests I see my family doctor - "That life should not be so hard."
I start Zoloft in August. It is not what I wanted to do. But the doctor explains that perhaps there is a chemical imbalance that is "physically depressing" my whole body function. It will take a few weeks to see if the Zoloft will help.

Mama's death is in September.

Zoloft does help with the control of my body. The physical strength of my body seemed to be hampered by how the brain was getting its signals. I am now tired at the end of the day from physical, not mental processing.

October 8th, a bad day of vertigo - when the room spins around you! I feel separated again. An increase in Zoloft is ordered.

Here I am! The walls are down!

In 1990 my daughter had given me a journal for my birthday with this inscription:

"Take some time, sit down, and record some of the wonderful ideas and philosophies you have."
                              Love always

Cassie

I realize now, that I am facing my own mortality. I won't always be here to share my life, my ideas. What will I leave behind? A bit of me. I find the journal.

Journal...
  No one is perfect.
  Build on the positive, not the negative.

Talents
  Everyone has natural talents... Something that is to them so easily achieved that they do not see it as special. It is the duty of a parent, friend or family to make sure that each person realizes their talents. We have a very hard time seeing our own talents because they come easily and naturally, hidden in our everyday actions. And yet it is what we can best give to society. So comes the need to be recognized, cultured and given direction.

Attitude

A positive attitude is 90% towards achieving. When life throws its blows, get right back up - don't dwell on them - look forward to the next step. Today is a new day. You can get dragged under in just 48 hours if you dwell on the negative. Let the blows roll off your back. Soak up all the good things - don't complain. You can achieve!

Children

As our children grow, we see them as a combination of all years past. We look and see the tiny infant first placed in our arms, the 18 month old becoming an individual and on... the ages and years
all combined - 6 years, 10 years, teens.
So when you grow up and feel we are not treating you of the age you are now, today; remember, to us, we still see the little one in you.
It is special because we are able to love all of you,
Always
With no questions.

Complete
My life has been truly full - I want for nothing more
than I have - because I have the greatest...
A husband whose love is never ending, never
questioning - strong. And two of the most beautiful
children created - I am so proud, they are the best.
They will survive.

1994
I have been given the chance to survive. To do this
I feel I need to make things simple and clear, I strive
for order - to surround myself with nature. I seem to
have lost my "German clutter" as my daughter calls
my decorating. I'd like to tear down the whole house.
But I'll start room by room.
This will give me more energy.
I must be getting better - for years I could not even
think of what I wanted, or needed to do with the house.

Smile
Give yourself a lift...
Smile at yourself in the mirror.
You are your own best friend.

Maturity

Maturity progresses in steps. When two people in a relationship are on the same level - all is harmony.
When one progresses several steps ahead it causes some upheaval.
Patience... usually the other will catch up and Harmony will prevail.

Life and Death

Life and death are the greatest challenges of a lifetime. In facing death, be it from war or illness, changes occur. You have to come to terms with it.
It is a step that takes you very far from your partner.
And your partner is struggling with the loss of the one they love, having to deal with a life apart.

When the war is over, or the illness cured, huge changes must occur. The partner who was struggling with the possible loss is ready to continue a life together because the threat is gone.
But the one who faced death has to now relearn how to face life (accept LIFE). Relearn that there is a future.

My husband and I have been on both sides.
Now we are back on the same step.

Masters of Wit

My Child
A Twinkle of the Eye
An Eyebrow raised in Response
Knowing Eyes scan ready

The Signal to Start
An innocent Question proposed
Wilily Answered, Ricocheted

Words quickly Juggled and Tossed
Patternless designs cleverly Diverted
Ingenuous notions of Success

Animated Jesting abounds
Intelligent Nonsense applauded
Pulling Others in...   Beware

"Got ya!" It's all on You
Laughter flowing, Bellies aching
Salty Tears streaming

Enjoy...
A Tickling of the Mind
Masters of Wit

Embarrassing...

My family and I are sitting in a local pizza restaurant. My tremors and jerks are at their peak. As a group of people walk by, my fork suddenly flies out of my hand and lands prongs down within inches of a lady's foot! She did not see what had happened - but my family did! They start laughing - making remarks about my table manners. I am so very upset, I could have hurt someone with my fork!! How could I have explained that one? We share the laughter together, the only way to get through the embarrassing moments!

I also inform my family that I will not get upset if they see things in our home that should be changed: like old food in the refrigerator or clothes that I should not wear. The only room that is off limits is the room with my medical research. I know that the room is a total mess, papers spread all over; but, I need it that way to think. If I file them neatly in a box, I will never remember where or what is there.

If I am on the same road as my mother and aunt, then I want to make it as easy as I can on my family. I will try not to have a "bad personality." (This, however, is not always in my control.)

Relearn to Read...

They cannot not be simple, the books I will use to relearn to read. My brain is no longer simple. I get lost in simple. Simple means one straight line from one idea to another. I have no straight lines left. My brain is working in alternate routes. Routes that go around, double back, split in two, rejoin, and finally reach where I want to go. I am speaking in abstract, descriptive phrases for single words. It has become a game for all who have the patience to listen to me. What is she trying to say now?

So I get lost in simple reading. Trying over and over to remember what I have just read. Trying over and over to comprehend what I have just read. The ideas end up on a dead end road.

And then I saw a review on TV about Dickens', *David Copperfield.* The language intrigues me. The "backward flowing" of early English reminds me of my own thought process.

So out comes Dickens, the earlier the better. I find it to be easier to follow. Not easy, but easier. For even then I am rereading and rereading - first paragraphs and then pages. But after a few hard weeks it starts to work. I no longer have to review what I have read before to follow the book.

I never was a "reader." Perhaps growing up on a farm we didn't have the quiet time to read. Although books were always there. We all had library cards. My fondest memories are going to the library with Mama and siblings in the summer. The great marble pillars, the high steps, smell of glue, leather and books. The "noisy" quiet of books banging, pages flipping, muffled coughs and whispers, dust collecting. Coming home with a pile of books little arms could hardly carry.

The "books" say when you relearn a task you learn it at a higher level. This proves to be very true. Simple "pages a day" turn into "chapters a day." I am so impressed. How is it I am reading better than I ever have? How is it after losing so much, I can regain at a much higher level? Will I be able to hold onto it? Will I remember?

And so I vow to read all of Dickens, taking as much time as needed.

Looking back, Dickens proves to be my best choice because as his books progress, he loses the "old English" style. The ending books are written quite "normal." So too, I have led my brain into a more "normal" way of thinking. It will take another four years of ups and downs to reach the point of no longer constantly talking in riddles, but I am headed in the right direction.

If I can have success in relearning to read, then maybe I can do more. Maybe I can stay ahead of this disease long enough for someone to find a cure...

July 1996

The first half of the year has gone well. Feeling good, energy up, keep on going, in control, smile easily, actually laugh out loud! Hand tremors, but not excessive. Night sweats, nightly. Twice in early July I feel dizzy - but after laying down, I am better. The morning of July 20th I have a bad spell of vertigo that lasts until 2:00 pm. I think, "Well, I'm on the blood pressure medicine and Zoloft, can't do anything about it - just go with it." I seem OK the rest of the day, so I forget it happened.

We are at a family event on August 4th, it is hot and humid. I tell my sisters, "I have not been feeling right the last two weeks. I can't take getting old this young." I ask my husband to take me home and I'm in bed by 5:00.

Thoughts: I feel a wave come over me - flat and thick. I follow it in, adjusting my breathing, the slower my breathing the deeper I go. I am not afraid. As I go deeper, I feel that it would be so easy to stop breathing and all would be over. I think about my family and maybe it would be better this way, Mama's death was so horrible. Not now. I get out of bed. Get back in control.

August 6th. I feel the walls trying to go up - stop - fight! I call my family doctor to see if I might need more Zoloft. I tell her I didn't feel right for the last two weeks, tremors are now the worst they have ever been. She asks how soon I could get into the University. Too long to wait. She makes appoint-ments with a local neurologist and a neuropsychologist.

AND THEN I REMEMBER THE VERTIGO

Analysis of the last two weeks:

> *Headache all the time like a strong pressure which is more severe in the back of my head on the right neck area and behind my right eye.
>
> *Dropping things every day.
>
> *In talking, words that I don't take the time to think about come out mixed up - with the syllables of one word put into another word.
>
> *Have to concentrate more on what I say
>
> *Tremors are constant in hands, arms, legs, and body.
>
> *Grinding feeling in right hand and right foot.
>
> *Some jerks, full movement of hands leading to dropping something or hitting my hand.

As the days follow, the tremors ease but pain sets in, along with a notable weakness. A gallon of milk is too heavy to lift.

The local neurologist and neuropsychologist don't have any new answers. They both suggest I go back to the University because that's where my baseline tests are.

The neuropsychologist did add that it is OK to be concerned. HE SEES SOMETHING IS WRONG. This is the first time I feel I am not "crazy" or "obsessed." We take with us information on a familial Alzheimer's Disease Research Center in the state of Washington.

The follow-up appointment at the University is in November.

October 20, 1996
"Do less now, so you can do more later."
I sit beside my frail Uncle in a darkened hospital room. A
small light casts a glow across his tired face. I gently rub his
forehead. Another vigil of death. Family members wait
down the hall, gathered in a quiet room. An Uncle with no
children of his own, we have a special bond, as he treated
us each as his own.

He has not spoken for hours, we again watch for signs of
discomfort - the unspoken word. As I lean over and whisper
a word of love, he responds with a very clear, "Do less now,
so you can do more later." His last words to me. Words that
I know have come straight from my mother, through him.
The door of death has already opened, he lay between two
worlds. Knowing of both worlds.

I ponder his words because up to now I have been
aggressively trying to maintain my "normal" activities. I have
not had the desire to "slow down" and I push until I drop.
It's the very Western way - if you don't use it, you'll lose it.
And I'll do anything to keep from losing more!

So what is this "Do less now..."?
Purposely slow down?
Perhaps he means if I slow down I can pace my energy out
over more years. I would be happy with more "normal"
years. The message is very strong and clear so I decide to
do my best to follow it.

November 6, 1996
I need to get to the University, a two hour drive. My tests are tomorrow, all day. I have always taken our Lumina van. I sit up high, it has a large sloping windshield and a good view. All day, it nags at me to take the station wagon. I decide to follow my instincts.

I'm about two thirds of the way there. It has become very dark, as night comes early this time of the year. All of a sudden in my headlights stands a large buck deer, body across my path, head with a full rack of horns turned looking straight at me, eyes fixed on the lights. There is not enough time to stop...

I am in a cocoon of air, as thick as pudding, surrounding me in a protective sea. We hit. I only feel a cushioned impact. I pull over to a stop. A lady behind me also stops. She said she never saw anything like it. The deer went flying over the top of the car, off to the left. The front end of the car is smashed, along with fur on the drivers side door handle. How is it I'm not hurt she asks?

If I had been in the van, the deer would probably have slid up the sloping hood and landed in my lap.

The protective force that I feel radiates the *spirits* of my Mother and Uncle.
I embrace this very *tangible* feeling.
They are showing me their strength.
Their love...

Thoughts...

It is in the 1970's. My Grandmother has passed away and my parents are fixing up the big farm house to move into. My mother has chosen wallpaper for the dinning room and has asked me to hang It for her. She Is In the kItchen, a separate room with a single doorway between. I am high on a ladder in a corner trying to cut the wallpaper to fit around the ornate wood trim. I am a bit frustrated. That room alone has two large banks of windows and six doors all surrounded by ornate wood trim. I'm working on the left side of the window, so my right hand is on top of my left, and I'm all twisted about up on the ladder when... my name is called out as clear as can be..."ChrIstIne"... wIth the emphasIs on "–tine." I turn from my project expecting to see my mother. The room is empty. First shock, and then a calm, as I realize it is my Grandmother. I have this overwhelming feeling that she is telling me she is pleased with what we are doing to her house. And then she is gone...

As more and more of my "active, everyday" brain closes down, the psychic side grows stronger. Perhaps it has always been there, but the everyday life and reality keep it from being heard. I would call it ESP, or tell our children all mothers have "eyes in the back of their heads." I would tease at work when a shipment of 15 boxes would arrive and a customer wanted a particular item. I was able to go to the box it was in. At my "best" I could visualize the people packing the boxes. And that would feel like time travel.

When our children moved from home to go to college, there would be nights I was up in a fearful, cold sweat knowing something was wrong. In the morning, talking to them over the phone, I'd find I had reason to be upset. But I wouldn't think much of it, we are a close family.

I have researched it more because it has happened so much more since my mother has passed. I do realize she is on a mission to make sure her family is safe and will not have to go through all that she did.

Also, it is important to realize early on that **healing** is supported through dreams, coincidences, déjà vu, intuition and other psychic possibilities.

Second Sight by Judith Orloff, MD explores the mystery of psychic gifts. It is her life story, but also gives a good understanding to what we all can feel. And that it is OK to feel it.

SECOND SIGHT by Judith Orloff, MD
Copyright © 1996 by Judith Orloff.
By permission of Warner Books, Inc.

Chapter 1   Children with psychic abilities who were not educated about them were prone to making preposterous assumptions about themselves. Everybody has such sensitivities but because of parents, teachers, or therapists they may be discounted or rejected. It takes immense energy to keep anything so powerful sealed up within, resulting in depletion and depression.

Chapter 2   Psychics often perceive many of the physical symptoms in the people around them. This powerful form of empathy, if unrecognized, could be overwhelming. Psychics must relax and let those perceptions flow right through them.
*Near-death experiences reinforce the idea that death is not an end but simply a transition into another form.
*Human beings are blessed with gifts never dreamed possible of which psychic ability is one.

Chapters 3 to 6 A personal journey

Chapter 7   The bedrock of spirituality is to learn about love.
*As a child psychic experiences may be frightening, to proceed, we must feel safe, we must know there is a net beneath us. Clarifying and strengthening spiritual beliefs is one way of providing that net. The form of spirituality can be traditional religion or not. The path needs to be compassionate, not based on power.
*This journey is open for all. Once you are ready to take a second look, to open the door a crack and reevaluate, everything is possible.

*The psychic flourishes when you give it space to grow. Meditation can provide this space.

Chapter 8   Dreams fall into two major categories: psychological and psychic. Psychological dreams deal with themes aimed at identifying and sorting through unclear emotions. Psychic dreams can give guidance, can be precognitive (dealing with the future), or healing.

Guidance dreams: You begin to expand your options by recognizing the refined interplay between the guidance received in dreams and your waking awareness.

*Dreams present possibilities that your intellect has not considered. Dreams can clarify your choices.

*The best approach is to write down a specific request on a piece of paper and place it next to your bed. In the morning, record your dreams and look to them for the answer. It may take several nights, or a combination of all nights.

*In analyzing guidance dreams look for intuitive clues, certain material that zings with energy and grabs your attention. Stay aware of your body's responses - goose bumps, a chill, flushing, etc. Perhaps you will have a very distinct "Ah-ha" feeling.

*Guidance dreams can often be red flags warning of danger. They can specifically tell you how and when to avoid danger.

*When the body is in a weakened state, the mind is less

chaotic and more susceptible to dreams.

Precognitive dreams: Clues to a precognitive dream include: startlingly vivid imagery, watching an event unfold that might be totally unrelated to you, being given information about your own future, waking up knowing details about events that have not yet occurred, or clarifying times, dates, places, or the direction your life is going to take.

*Precognitive dreams can set you on a particular path, it is your responsibility to carry out that goal.

*They are evidence of the depth of connection we can have with the world around us.

*In intuitive states, past, present, and future blur together in a continuum. Looking into the future is the same as the present or past.

Healing dreams: There is a healing instinct within us that can manifest itself in our dreams. When you are asleep you open yourself up to healing forces.

*In dreams, resistances and inhibitions fall away; things can happen that you don't ordinarily give yourself permission to experience.

*Your dreams can be with you every step of the process - from the initial diagnostic phase and through treatment.

*They may even enable you to find a cure.

*Although some premonitions can be painful to accept, they're actually special gifts. If you detect an illness in the early stages or seek treatment soon enough to prevent its spread, you may avoid undue suffering.

*As significant as dreams are that guide you to healing, there are those that themselves have the power to do the healing. We all are capable of dreams that heal the body.

*When you dream you merge with a benevolent intelligence that touches you, and in some special circumstances it even heals.

*Attend to your dreams.

*Give yourself a chance to learn from them.

Dream Journals: The real art of dreaming is in remembering our dreams. Dream journals allow us to honor our inner lives, and are a living testament to our personal odysseys.

*In keeping a dream journal, we not only chronicle the patterns of our unconscious, we can also begin to pinpoint and make use of our psychic dreams. Our journals play a dynamic role.

*They house the psychic guidance we request to live our lives well so the knowledge we gain can't be lost, misinterpreted, or forgotten.

*They're a living testament to the healing we receive in dreams, so that we can remember and make full use of this healing.

*Containing concrete evidence of our future predictions, our journals enable us to correlate our dreams with an actual event when it takes place.

Chapter 9   Synchronicities: inspired coincidences viewed as other than haphazard events with an acknowledgement that a greater force is moving through our lives linking us all together.

*Déjà vu: the sense of having been somewhere or known someone before.

*Clairvoyance: psychically picking up an event as it is actually happening.

*Precognition, when you accurately predict an event before it occurs.

*Prescience, a psychic empathy where you seem to take on other people's moods or even feel their physical symptoms, "overly sensitive."

Chapter 10   The well-balanced psychic uses her gift discerningly, radiating an understated sense of calm.

*Psychic abilities can be learned or be a natural evolution of spiritual growth. Over-thinking kills creativity, as it does the psychic.

*The magic comes when you give up mental control and allow a greater force to take hold. In this groove you can be showered with original ideas and intuitive insights.

*The intensity of the creative process, the surrender required to get to the really good stuff inside, is exactly what fuels the psychic. Just as the psychic ebbs and flows, so do rhythms and cycles of the creative. Take time to relax, allowing the gained wisdom gained to incubate.

Chapter 11   Our task is to solidify our connection with a higher power through meditation or prayer, and to make love a priority in how we think and behave. We're the template for where love begins. The more we love and accept ourselves, the more we're able to love and accept other people. To be psychic can be our entry into a full-bodied spiritual life, where love abides and everything has a purpose. Love gives us the power to transform any seeming calamity into an asset and source of comfort.

Chapter 12   Imagine what the world would be like if children were praised and encouraged to voice their psychic abilities instead of being stigmatized, discounted, or judged. Imagine a whole generation growing up more balanced and happy, expressing their gift, not being pressured into pretending to be something they're not.
*Beyond technology, beyond the grandest achievements of the intellectual mind, our bodies and spirits are aching to be healed, physically as well as spiritually.
*When science and spirituality finally join forces, medicine will achieve its full power. And doctors, by reviving their own spirits, will become true healers once again.
*Our healing comes from the flow of love as we reach out to others, in the simplest of actions: a word of encouragement, a smile, or a pointed question at the right time is all that's required.

November 27, 1996

The report back from the University neuropsychologist once again puts the emphasis of any changes onto depression. Why is it that they cannot see what is happening? Why is it "they" feel everyone has to fit into a pigeon hole and if they don't know what is happening it is so much easier to put on a label than to say, "At this time we don't know, but we are concerned and will listen to you"? The report does not even have all the basic facts right! How can they do such a bad job? What about the person who no longer can speak out? I should not have been surprised, Mama's neuropsychological reports were not any more definitive, even when she was very Ill.

But because of the changes in the tests on motor/muscle performance, Dr. Brooks, Neurology University of WI, Madison prescribes Amantadine, a Parkinson medication. The symptoms are Parkinsonian in nature. The episodes of vertigo could be associated with changes in the temporal lobe. Depression, however, is given equal consideration.

Had Dr. Brooks and his team not developed the fine motor/ muscle evaluation tests, there would be no way to see that I was physically slipping... Up to now, Alzheimer's Disease is only rated by dementia through the neuropsychologists and you almost have to be at the "unfunctioning" level... and then it is too late.

And anyway, there is no treatment yet.

Another MRI is ordered.

November 1996
Following the advice of our local neuropsychologist, I
contact the Alzheimer's Disease Research Center, University
of Washington State. They take down our family medical
information.

At this time, the family is too small for their current genetic
research. The family information is kept in their files. I am
asked to contact them when a clearer picture of my health
condition is known, or if other family members are affected.
They are, however, very interested.
They supply an 800 number where I can reach them.
I need more proof...   How can I get it?...

I also contact the Alzheimer's National Chapter and am sent
current studies. There are six main ones. I am very excited
when the papers arrive. Maybe I can enter a study and
move ahead on finding an answer. It is disappointing when
I realize that at this time there are not any that I fit into,
mostly I am too young...

I always thought we were very lucky and special to be able to grow up on a farm. I think it is the land that I liked the best. As children we had fields and fields to roam unlike the children in town who only had their back yards. I appreciated it even more after I was married and moved into the city and adjusted to my own "back yard."

Celestine Prophecy by James Redfield 1993 (published by Warner Books) addresses that energy which we as children felt but did not understand.

Finding meditative "Bliss" and entering that state to heal is an integral part of the overall healing process. James Redfield takes me to a place which I can readily reenter to feel the bliss and energy. Just as I did as a child. He puts into words the "vision of bliss" which up to now was only an idea I had read about in multiple books.

James Redfield follows with three more books, each going one step further into the process of utilizing energy, intuition and the coincidences about us.

For me, his books add to my very foundation for healing.

I pick up the book *Parkinson's Disease* by Abraham
Lieberman, MD and Frank Williams 1993, Published by
Simon & Schuster, A Fireside Book.
It gives me a basis for the Parkinsonian symptoms and the
uses of the medications. It is helpful in understanding
some of the symptoms and which ones do not fit into this
profile. There is also a chapter on *Planning Your Financial
Future* that is very straightforward.

Financial Planning....
I don't know how fast this will go. If I can lose so much in
such a short time how long will I be able to function? How
soon will I need help?

With Mama, all went before we could accept it. Each trip to
the University we were sure there would be answers. And
then it was too late. She could no longer think for herself,
she could no longer communicate. We found our family
sitting before a judge. He tried to be understanding, but
how do you pronounce a woman, the one who once was the
strength of a family, now incompetent without hurting those
before him?

My husband and I choose to face this early. The correct
papers are drawn up in the lawyers office. The pain is still
there. But we are able to share it as a couple...
To hold each other and grieve.

Maybe... Hopefully... the papers will not be needed soon.

A Partnership...

I remember back to taking our daughter to the doctor when she was in Jr. High School. The nurse ushered us into an examination room and said, "Have a seat, the doctor will be right in." Our daughter went right for the "doctor stool" and sat down. I'm looking at this and deciding whether to say anything. On the one hand, I've been raised with a strict sense of authority. Is this a demonstration of "lack of authority/respect?" On the other side, I'm proud that she is relaxed enough to see the doctor as a friend. Perhaps she may be a doctor, herself, one day.

I often look back on that day as I am thrown into the "patient" chair quite often these days. If healing is to work, I need not put the doctors onto an infallible pedestal. This is a partnership. We each have equal information to share.

Finding a cure or healing is as much, or more, my responsibility than the doctors'. I am aware of what is happening to me and without this information the doctors will not have a clue as to what is wrong or more importantly - what is working. The doctors have their medical knowledge to share with me. With this knowledge, I can add to the self-healing powers within and about me.

Together we can make it happen.

Journal...

Not Special
  Be content and proud of the little things you do each
  day. They may not seem that grand at the time, but
  in looking back each has piled up to be extra-ordinary!
  Painting a wall or fixing a closet door - in the end you
  have a beautiful house. Or starting a business and
  running it day after day - in the end you have lived fine,
  employed others who have lived fine, satisfied (or not)
  thousands of people - and have something left.
  And it just didn't seem like anything special at the time.

Old
  Today I see you no longer as a child of mine made up
  of years being a child. Today I called you "old" -
  Why was that?
  Today I see you as an adult - one who is stronger
  than I.
  The roles are reversing.

Thank you
  Thank you, family, for always being here and
  not letting me pull you down -
  Keep smiling!

A Visit to a Nursing Home

Fragmented Bodies
Next to Fragmented Minds
Locked in
Each holding the oneness
    Of the Other

Together they could be
    Whole
Unknowing next to knowing
Unwalking next to walking

Separate souls on one
    Journey
Joined by shared
    Fragmentation
All awaiting Distant Shores

This is the hardest chapter to write. The changes are severe.

We started our current business in 1985. After a job change for my husband, he was looking for something new. When traveling for his old job, he stopped to visit an old landlord from his college years. The landlord now ran a hobby store. We decided to research the idea along with including science items. Our son was very interested in science and we were having a hard time finding supplies. It had been our plan for me to hold another paying job and my husband to work the store until the store was productive. However, right before we were ready to open, he received a job offer he could not refuse. I ran the store in the daytime and he took over late in the afternoon and weekends. I learned very quickly to read product brochures upside down as I gave my "sales pitch" on the products I knew nothing about! Men were not used to seeing women working in hobby stores, so as the years went by, they would come in, direct their questions to one of the sales clerks next to me, who would then turn to me for the answers. It was always a standing joke among us.

Our store was located across the street from my parent's home. As my mother became more ill, I became a fast back-up for my Dad. While she was still able to walk, he would drop her by and she would sit quietly in the office. When she lost her ability to walk, I could easily run across to them.

And then all changed...

I started leaving my customers to find some product information for them and never returning because I was asked a question by an employee, or had to answer the phone and forgot they were there. Or I'd be in the middle of a "sales pitch" about the product and suddenly forget everything - having to hand them over to another clerk. I went very quickly from knowing every part of the business, including information on over 14,000 different items, to nothing...

My husband had to give up his job as I became more ill and less able to work. The physical pain, tremors and lack of strength continued to worsen.... And with it the amount of time that I was able to stay at the store.

January 1997

I have not been taking prescription drugs very much of my life - only most recently - so when I pick up my refill of amantadine and it is totally a different color I "obey" them and take it. It is a different brand; "same thing" I am told. I decide to try the "new" red one before I run out of the other yellow ones. Within a very short time (hours) I am experiencing difficulty breathing, dizziness, and a tightness in my chest. I call the University and am told to only take the yellow amantadine. At the pharmacy, they said some people are allergic to the yellow and some are allergic to the red. I am told that with such a severe reaction I should never try the red again. "Don't even touch it" is their advice!

Why then did they switch me? And why wasn't this given out in the information with the prescription? And how could anyone taking care of someone else possibly know all this?

I go back through our mother's medication list. I remember the University trying several different drugs. In finding her medication (Papa saved a little of each tried, with a note on what didn't work) I see she was given RED amantadine. It was given only for a very short time, with bad side affects. We were never told there was a YELLOW amantadine. Maybe she did not have to suffer so much...

I can only believe she is watching out for me and saw that the pharmacist filled my first prescription with YELLOW... How else? They said the red was more common... although the name brand is yellow.

January 1997

The end of January brings another visit to the University. The amantadine has been successful in relieving a lot of pain while the drug is in effect - about four hours. The test results show the tremors have increased and my strength has continued to decrease. Eldepryl is added in for the episodes of confusion and weakness. When I have the prescription filled the pharmacy questions a possible interaction with Zoloft.

As I have stopped driving out of town, our son and his fiancée drove me to the University with a mutual promise of being able to shop in the unique shops about town. I didn't expect to find any particular items, so I was merely browsing; enjoying the old buildings, uneven wood floors, college atmosphere, and Eastern cultures. However, the very first book I picked off a shelf tucked in a corner proved to hold the answers to so many of my questions. "Stress and cortisol" were words that caught my attention. The tremors alone have added stress to my life. If I come under high stress it may take days for me to "calm back down." As when taking the tests at the University. I will be sick for days after, unable to slow my brain down enough to sleep.

Brain Longevity The Breakthrough Medical Program That Improves Your Mind and Memory by Dharma Singh Khalsa, M.D. is the book for my library. Dr. Khalsa has focused his career on finding the "cortisol connection" to neurological degeneration. He has developed a treatment program that is patient based.

April 1997

The episodes of vertigo are increasing. April brings an episode of tachycardia, shortness of breath and systolic and diastolic hypertension (panic attacks). My sister takes me down to the University for an unscheduled check-up. She knows something is very wrong. Hyperserotonin syndrome is suspected because of the inter action between Zoloft and Eldepryl. I am to stop the Eldepryl and reduce the Amantadine. By the 24th of the month I have pain, hurt, grinding tremors, cannot think, cannot sequence, cannot add, it is hard to complete sentences, more pain, hard to walk... CRASH... scream, dropping things... Pain.

We are supposed to go on a business trip in three days. I'll never make it! In reading *Brain Longevity,* Dharma Singh Khalsa, M.D. addresses Eldepryl (Deprenyl) in the chapter on pharmacology. He states that Eldepryl has been used in Europe for many years to treat depression and cognitive decline. So maybe I would not need both Zoloft and Eldepryl. I decide to try the Eldepryl and Amantadine again and drop the Zoloft. It takes a full month to achieve the proper balance, but I feel this is a much better combination. The drawback to these medications is that they wear off before the day is out. So although it is helping, I am still limited to a four hour window, but at this point I will take what I can get.

I am excited about the information in *Brain Longevity.* Dr. Khalsa is very thorough, this is one book that could be read cover to cover.

Chapter 1

Alzheimer's Disease can be delayed and prevented.
Age-associated memory impairment can be eradicated.
People in their forties, fifties, sixties - and beyond - can
retain not only an almost perfect memory, but can also
have "youthful minds," characterized by the dynamic
brain power, learning ability, creativity, and emotional
zest usually found only in young people. This program,
that is at the white-hot forefront of anti-aging medicine,
employs complementary medicine.

Alzheimer's is a mental condition characterized by
extensive death of brain cells. Based upon research and
clinical work, excessive cortisol production is one of the
primary causes of death of those cells. The other causes
appear to be genetic factors, environmental factors,
metabolic factors, and decreased blood flow to the brain.

Excess cortisol is causing a decline in the day-to-day
function of the brain. Cortisol robs the brain of its only
source of fuel: glucose. It also wreaks havoc on the
brain's chemical messengers, the neurotransmitters,
which carry your thoughts from one brain cell to the next.

Until not long ago, researchers thought the brain was essentially static, that once damage was done, it couldn't be undone. But all the new technology of the past few decades, such as CAT, PET, and MRI, has shown that because of the brain's unique regenerative power, "brain plasticity," blighted areas of the brain can be brought back to life. The brain doesn't store each of its memories in single, separate brain cells or neurons. Memories exist in networks of connected neurons. If one neuron is killed, the brain can switch its memory connection through another neuron; this is redundant circuitry. Neurons are 60% fat.

Western medicine constantly strives to reduce each illness to a specific, isolated cause with a single "magic bullet" cure. Most degenerative diseases, including Alzheimer's, have a number of different causes, and may have different causes in different people. Thus the need for a multi-factorial treatment program. Dr. Khalsa's program includes nutritional therapy; supplementation with specific vitamins, minerals, and trace elements; administration of natural medicinal tonics; cardiovascular exercise; mental exercise; yogic mind/body exercises; stress management; and certain pharmaceutical medications. People with very mild cognitive impairment, or no cognitive impairment, have used the mental fitness program to develop minds that can focus and learn with incredible efficiency. It has also worked miracles for accident victims with brain damage who were supposedly beyond the help of medicine. Many things that help the brain to regenerate also help the rest of the body to restore itself. The healing comes from within. Age-associated memory impairment and early-stage Alzheimer's Disease are often linked. The primary clinical goal is to intervene in the earliest possible stages of cognitive decline. It is much easier to prevent cognitive decline than to reverse it. This is not a "cure" for Alzheimer's, but a slowing of the progression. In delaying, we may be able to spare patients from the worst advanced stages.

Chapter 2

The people rescued from Alzheimer's will also experience a very positive phenomenon. They won't grow less intelligent as they age; they'll just grow wiser. Their ever-increasing neuronal branches will give them a rich, complex sense of understanding. Their vast experience will endow them with a deep, abiding comprehension of life.

Robert Sapolsky, PhD of Stanford University writes: There are three essential ways that stress destroys optimal function of the brain and blots out memory.
* First, when cortisol is released in a stressful situation, it

inhibits the utilization of blood sugar by the brain's primary memory center, the hippocampus. The brain is unable to lay down a memory.

* Second, cortisol overproduction interferes with the function of the brain's neurotransmitters so even if a memory has been laid down in the past it can no longer be easily accessed.

* Third, too much cortisol kills brain cells by disrupting brain cell metabolism and causing excessive amounts of calcium to enter brain cells producing free radicals.

To reduce stress all people must find their own balance between mental and physical work and their energy level. And they must then maintain it.

Dr. Khalsa's program is characterized by simplicity and common sense as it is a lifestyle program - not a "magic bullet" treatment - which is relatively more patient-managed than physician-managed. Each patient is ultimately responsible for his or her own healing; all a doctor can do is inaugurate and monitor the process. The program is broad based with a general pro-health function rather than a specific anti-disease function. This encourages activation of self-healing powers.

Nutritional therapy can help repair damaged neurons, protect neurons and neurotransmitters from further damage, and improve day-to-day biochemical function in even a damaged brain. "What's good for the heart is good for the head." The brain requires about 25 percent of all blood pumped by the heart. A "nutrient dense" low-fat diet, high in complex carbohydrates, with adequate protein, delivering high amounts of key nutrients, while causing minimal stress upon organs of digestion and assimilation will also stabilize blood sugar levels. Blood sugar is the only source of fuel for the brain. Stress increases nutritional needs so people under high stress require extra nutrients.

It is critically important to reduce stress levels. The more damage to the brain a person has suffered, the harder it is to "turn off" stress. The physical effects of stress are greatly magnified when people feel "out of control." Stress that comes as a surprise evokes a much greater physical stress response. Most of the negative physical impact of stress can be avoided if a person doesn't "hold it in," or if there is a social support system from friends or family. Effort should be made to reduce the actual number of stressors. An extremely powerful tool against stress is meditation, in whatever form, including prayer. Stress is a highly subjective experience, and no method of managing it should be dismissed.

Dr. Khalsa has developed a series of yogic mind/body

exercises to increase mental fitness. These exercises restore the brain's biochemical ability to lay down new memories, and to focus intensely for extended periods, along with stimulating access to existing "remote" memories of long-past events. The sequence of specific movements are linked to a breathing pattern, a posture, and a mantra. These exercises drive nutrient-rich blood to the brain and to particular endocrine glands.

Another extremely important form of exercise is mental exercise. Just using the brain actually increases its size and also increases the number of dendritic branches of brain cells. Mental exercise can include anything from reading to playing cards to playing along with quiz shows on television.

Based upon clinical experience, as well as double-blind studies performed by many researchers, Dr. Khalsa has come to believe that Alzheimer's progression can be significantly retarded, in some cases, with vigorous pharmacological intervention. It also appears as if symptoms of early-stage age-associated memory impairment can often be completely eradicated with proper medication. Furthermore, certain medications help some patients without frank cognitive pathology to achieve very high levels of concentration, learning ability, and creativity. The brain longevity programs do not rely extensively upon the use of pharmaceutical drugs, but instead try to stimulate the patient's body to heal itself. The pharmaceutical agents are used more aggressively in the early phases of the patient's program and gradually lowered as their body and mind regain their former powers.

Parts Two and Three go into "How the Brain Works" and "Designing Your Own Brain Longevity Program" with specific information listed on supplements, meditation, exercises and pharmacology.

It is well worth reading this information as it is the most complete that I have been able to find, up to now.
* Dr. Khalsa stresses early intervention and prevention. Two words that have not yet made it into the main stream.
* He sets forth the terms "age associated memory impairment" and "mild cognitive impairment" which will not reach the researchers for several more years.
* He shares a complete listing of nutrition supplements, and pharmacology choices along with stress reducers, stimulating self-healing.

May 1997

I have to make a decision. I am unable to keep up with family and friends when shopping, day trips, etc. I can either not go or I can get a wheelchair for those days. I should not isolate myself. My sisters and I plan a weekend get away with our daughters. I borrow a wheelchair. It is harder than I expected to be pushed in a wheelchair - to have someone else in charge of your movements.
A "humbling experience..."

I'm standing before the mirror, applying my usual make-up, as I have for so many years. Only this time, when I am done, I do not recognize me as me. No matter what I try, I cannot achieve that "look" that I liked and always had. The change has been gradual - I kept thinking "next time I'll get it back," but now it is gone. I can no longer look at myself in the mirror... another adjustment... another loss...

I'm in the kitchen, it's breakfast. O.K., I certainly know how to cook eggs and toast!! Concentrate! The morning medications have not yet kicked in. The eggs are in the pan. The bread is in the toaster. Good.
What is that?   What is next?   Try harder!
The toast is burning... throw it away.
The eggs are done. Plate in one hand - lift out the eggs... onto the plate... a jerk of the hand - the eggs go onto the floor! Throw it all away.
Tears... Pain...

Why has it become so hard? I cannot accept this change.

June 1997

I'm sitting in a comfortable chaise lab chair similar to a dental chair, to my right is a bank of oscilloscopes, before me sits a smaller oscilloscope, and off to the left a computer. We are at the University Clinic starting off my appointment with the motor/muscle testing. The motor/muscle doctor patiently explains (as he does each time) that by attaching sensory electrodes with tape to various spots they are able to register types and intensity of tremors, and speed and strength of response to various physical activities. It is also explained that some of the earliest stages of some diseases will show up as loss of strength in the tongue, thus each of these fine measurements become extremely important to the bigger picture in the diagnosis of a disease. I can go into a doctor and say "I have what appears to be tremors." But with this testing they will know what type and the intensity of the tremors. I have been to other neurologists, but no one else was able to classify to this point.

Even more important is the ability to see if the medications and alternative nutrition therapies are working. Or what negative effect they may have long before more drastic damage is done.

Tremor types:

      Isometric: During submaximal force targeted contractions

      Rest: During awake, relaxed conditions

Posture: During sustained arm positions
Intention: End-point osciliation during finger to nose
     test
Action: Imposed continuously on movements

Tremors are registered through the jaw, tongue, upper extremity (hand), lower extremity (foot), and head.
I show several types of tremors: rest, postural, isometric, and intention. This suggests that both central and peripheral pathogenetic mechanisms are involved.

Today is an important test because, although I still feel tremors, the testing has shown significant improvements. Which may be due to the pharmacological therapy with Amantadine and Eldepryl.

It is a good sign of early intervention.
My sisters usually accompany me to my appointments, both because this is hereditary, and because I will not remember all of what is said. We often bring articles found on Alzheimer's. Dr. Brooks is very patient with our input.

Ibuprofen is added in as a possible delaying of any Alzheimer's type dementia.

A letter from my younger sister to our family:
June 9,1997

Dear Family
On June 4th, I accompanied Chris to her appointment at the
clinic, there was some very good news. All the struggling
Chris had since Jan. with her medications was finally seeing
some positive results, with the new combination she tried.
Stopping the Zoloft but continuing the Eldepryl and
Amantadine has resulted in her motor muscle strength
improving back to the ability she had in 1994. Which is
great because she had experienced a 45% decrease of
strength in 1996. Her blood pressure remains stable with
the Captopril and her tremors have also subsided
significantly. She also has been taking 3 doses of a good
multivitamin and mineral supplements daily. When Chris'
medicines wear off at night she does lose her strength and
ability to function, but there is nothing that can be done as
she is at the maximum dosage of these meds.

We had a very long and informative talk with Dr. Brooks.
He really takes the time with Chris, I believe because her
case is so unique and because he is so impressed with the
research she has done and how she diligently keeps track of
her daily symptoms - she had 8 pages of typed notes for him
since her last appointment.

Chris is willing to be used for a study but Dr. Brooks said she is just like Mom in that this illness is unique and does not meet the criteria for a dementia study conducted with the rest of the masses. But with the research that has been done on Alzheimer's it is clear that our family is at risk for dementia and each offspring of Mom should take the proven, effective steps in prevention:

*Two times per day take 200 mg of Ibuprofen with food. Ibuprofen is Advil, Motrin or Nuprin, not Tylenol or Aspirin. The Ibuprofen must be taken with food so there is no disturbance to the stomach lining.

*Estrogen replacement for menopausal women.

*Eliminate Aluminum in water, antiperspirants (deodorants free of aluminum are: Arm&Hammer stick deodorant with baking soda and Mennen Crystal Clean Deodorant by Lady Speed Stick), aluminum cookware, soft drinks, processed cheese, canned parmesan cheese, white self rising flour, baking soda, cake mixes, frozen dough, pancake mixes, table salt, antacids, and pickled vegetables.

*Increase your level of Zinc by taking a good multivitamin and mineral supplement daily no matter how good you may think you are eating.

*Fluoride water is good. Helps fight off aluminum in your body.

*Tobacco smoke and previous head injury puts you at a higher risk.

Dr. Brooks believes whole heartedly and follows the above
lifestyle for himself, except for the estrogen of course!!!
He said it was very important that I inform you and urge
you to do the same. I have attached documents that
support what he says that I had come across in my reading.
Also included is info on heart attack prevention; we also
could be at risk for this because of our genes.

The next appointment for Chris at the clinic is Nov. 26th.
We would be happy to discuss any questions or concerns
you may have, please let us know. We all should be grateful
that we have a sister who could easily give up but who
researches and daily logs her symptoms in an effort to figure
out anything she can to help herself and others who may
also become inflicted with this illness. It would be much
easier for her to give up than to fight; such strength as this,
we were taught by Mom when faced with her own illness.

So love, hugs and support for Chris' continued strength
and...
Great health to all.

Rosann

A trip to the bookstore... and sitting on a table in the aisle among other books... is *The Highly Sensitive Person* How to Thrive When the World Overwhelms You by Elaine N. Aron, Ph.D. Published by Broadway Books.

Dr. Aron addresses the issues of being sensitive which are over arousal and over stimulation, resulting in stress. This causes chemical changes, and adjustments. Being sensitive may be one more "environmental" factor in the brain damage due to chemical stress. I find the book most helpful in understanding the added stress of being sensitive... which I am.

The next book to give me some help is *Beyond Prozac Brain-Toxic Lifestyles, Natural Antidotes & New Generation Antidepressants* by Michael J. Norden, M.D., Published by Regan Books. 1996

I am most impressed by the basic information on the neurotransmitter, Serotonin .

Beyond Prozac Brain-Toxic Lifestyles, Natural Antidotes & New Generation Antidepressants
Michael J. Norden, M.D., Regan Books, HarperCollins
10 East 53rd Street, New York, NY 10022

*Since World War II, depression has been increasing across international, cultural, and ethnic boundaries.
*The neurotransmitter, serotonin, (neurotransmitters convey messages from cell to cell throughout the central nervous system) influences important aspects of physiology, including body temperature, blood pressure, blood clotting, immunity, pain, digestion, sleep, and daily body rhythms.
*Heat in the form of both high temperature and high humidity is associated with a decrease in serotonin (and dopamine) activity. Serotonin can be measured in the blood and in the brain. Rising *blood serotonin* causes more blood clotting which can lead to heart attack. When we raise *brain serotonin* function, *blood serotonin* decreases.

*Light therapy has increased serotonin and melatonin.

*The pineal gland converts serotonin to melatonin.

*Melatonin works with serotonin to help us adapt to basic environmental rhythms - day and night, shields against free radical damage to the DNA at the cell level, and increases the release of growth hormone.

*From the treadmill to any repetitive movement such as chewing gum, exercise stimulates an increase in serotonin.

*Vitamins (C, E, and B), minerals and amino acid supplements will aid in serotonin levels.

*The ingestion of artificial sweeteners with aspartame has been linked to increases in depression.

*Cholesterol makes more serotonin available in the nerve synapses. Low blood cholesterol levels result in greater rates of depression.

*The correct balance of 30 percent protein, 30 percent fat, and 40 percent carbohydrate in the diet will promote a balance of insulin and its balancer glucagon along with balancing the production of good prostaglandins (anti-inflammatory) opposed to the bad prostaglandins (inflammatory).

*Essential fatty acids (Omega 3's) should also be added to help this balance.

*Prostaglandins often control the release of serotonin. Serotonin in turn heavily influences the production of prostaglandins.

November 1997

University appointment.

Because of the family history of dementia and the recent article in JAMA (Journal of American Medical Association) regarding the potentially beneficial effects of **Ginkgo Biloba**, Dr. Brooks suggests adding this into my regimen along with **Vitamin E** at 800 IU per day and **Ibuprofen** at 800 mg per day. The Ibuprofen has shown in some studies to delay the onset of dementia. The JAMA report stated that Ginkgo Biloba has shown a positive effect on attention and performance in dementing disorders and may actually be able to delay the onset of some symptoms.

We also discuss American Ginseng for energy. There has also been a change in the blood pressure medicine.

We, as a family, are happy to have a doctor who is open to all strategies for prevention/intervention.

Vitamin E

Food sources: Vegetables - spinach, parsley, mustard,
sweet potato and turnip leaves. Apple skins, egg
yolk, fish, meat, almonds, peanuts.

Canning of food results in a 40 to 65% loss of vitamin E.
Freezing does not degrade vitamin E, but some
loss may occur during storage. Sun drying will
destroy 100%.

Vitamin E is sold as a natural or synthetic preparation.
Natural, unesterified , d-alpha tocopherol.
Synthetic, esterified dl-alpha-tocopherol, acetate or
succinate and alpha tocopheryl nicotinate.

The unesterified form is absorbed from the digestive tract,
the esterified forms need to be converted first.

Buy a good brand, as some of the processing can be toxic.

Vitamin C protects vitamin E as well as helps to
regenerate vitamin E. Use together.

Vitamin E and Zinc act to stabilize cellular membranes.

It increases the survival of nerve cells.

In combination with deprenyl it is researched to slow
down Parkinsonism.

Vitamin E is being used to prevent and in conjunction
with treatments for cancer.

It is being seen to prevent platelet aggregating (strokes).

A powerful antioxidant that prevents lipid oxidation.

Vitamin E improves oxygen utilization and enhances
immune responses.

Ginkgo Biloba A.K.A.,: Maidenhair Tree

Many European studies now support the benefits from Ginkgo Biloba that the people of Asia knew for thousands of years.

Ginkgo Biloba improves circulation throughout the body, increasing overall oxygen levels.

Cerebral (brain) circulation aids in improving memory loss, alertness, concentration, depression, headaches, dizziness, anxiety and vertigo.

Ginkgo Biloba increases levels of glucose and ATP, which help maintain energy levels within individual cells.

By stabilizing the membranes involved in the blood-brain barrier, less swelling (edema) and complete restoration of function can be expected following an injury.

Peripheral circulation aids in leg cramps, improved walking for peripheral vascular disease, and the hands benefit in Raynaud's Disease. The Germans also use it to treat varicose veins.

The oxygenation of the body will improve altitude sickness with the increased blood flow to the heart reducing shortness of breath.

The fragility of the capillaries is reduced preventing strokes. And the complication of strokes: memory, balance, vertigo and disturbed thought process is all improved.

Ginkgo Biloba holds important vascular effects by
lowering blood pressure and dilating peripheral
blood vessels, including capillaries without
sacrificing cerebral circulation.

May be one of the most effective drugs against migraines.

Ginkgo Biloba is the first choice for tinnitis (ringing in the
ears.) Has shown improvements in hearing loss.

Improved retina health brings better eyesight and
possible damage reversal in macular degeneration.

As an anti-oxidant, it demonstrates an ability to neutralize
free radicals.

Ginkgo Biloba increases dopamine synthesis,
acetylcholine, epinephrine and norepinephrine.
Aids in total reactivation of neuronal network.

Aids in both Alzheimer's and Parkinson's Disease.
Improvements in alertness, increase in vigilance,
and increases in the rate of information processing
at neuronal levels.

Patients suffering from acute and chronic hemorrhoids
have received great relief.

Ginkgo Biloba appears to be safe, well tolerated, and
results can be achieved even at very low doses.

As with all herbs, look for high quality supplements.

Entwined With Love

My Child
There are Vines Entwined
          In our Tree of Life
Touching where other Branches
          Cannot reach

Bringing Flowers and Fruits of
          Pleasure and Delight
Making our life Full and Complete

Always there with Strength
Coiled in Comfort

With Love...
Friends...
You

dreams…

> Early 1998
> I am standing on a set of boards
> that are stretched across a pit.
> As I move the boards adjust up and down.
> This is very unstable. I am unable to step off
> the boards to safety before…
> I fall.

I have this dream several times over the years.
As the time passes, however,
I am able to awake before I fall
And still later…
To step off to safety before I awake.

January 1998

I start out the year by summarizing where I am physically, socially, and mentally. It is a very hard process and takes weeks to complete. I have been trying all along to give an accurate report to the doctors, but obviously I am failing because they don't understand.

PHYSICAL:

   Now:

        Standing limited to 5 - 10 minutes

        Walking limited to 2 - 3 blocks

        Low level of strength

             Hard to roll up car windows

             Hard to open aspirin bottles

             1 quart liquid maximum to carry

             2 plates maximum to carry

             Prefer paperbacks to hardcover books for
                  weight

             Unable to pull weeds or dig to plant bulbs

        Tremors

             Cannot draw a straight line

             Fingers tremor and repeat letters in typing

             Cannot carry a cup upon a saucer

             Cannot safely pour coffee

             Hard to eat soup

             Difficulty in cooking

        Extreme fatigue when medication wears off - 4 hour
                  maximum

        Extreme dry mouth in nervous situations

        Pain throughout my body

Depression - unable to take Prozac or Zoloft as it affects other medications.

MEALS

Used to:

Shopped, planned, and cooked 90% of all meals.

Had meals in slow cooker before going to work

Cooked meals from start to finish in less than 1 hour.

Canned and froze foods, and made jams and sauces.

Made specialty foods.

Now:

Husband has taken over the grocery shopping.

Make myself breakfast and 1 to 3 other meals per week.

Eat out or carry in rest of meals.

Easily emotional blow up if I push to make a meal.

Burn myself on oven or steam, cut myself, drop a lot of items including full plates of food, break dishes.

Cannot do two tasks at the same time.

Have made a list of food and what I can cook because I cannot remember.

DRIVING:

Used to:

Drive all over the state and country

Now:

Uncomfortable to drive more than 30 miles

Uncomfortable to drive at night

Cannot scrape icy windows until after defroster has melted all the ice

WORK:

Used to:

Work 8+ hour days

Worked on the sales floor, bookkeeping, ordering, and payroll

Was out-going and a pleasant, people person

Now:

No longer able to handle daily situations

Cannot answer multiple questions of customers or employees

Unable to determine long-term outcomes to decisions

Get emotionally upset in new settings

Get emotionally upset with changes - computer, tax forms

Paranoid over staff doing their job

Fly off in temper in inappropriate situations

Unable to make decisions, even simple - What to do with mail?

Hard to smile when with customers giving information

Cannot find my physical space - bump into walls, displays, and run over children

Have had to hire replacements for my jobs

Only working over lunch hour for relief of husband

Cannot work alone

HOUSEWORK:
> Used to:
>> Did all house, yard, gardening, painting, wall-papering - inside and out
>
> Now:
>> Have a cleaning person come once a week for all cleaning
>>
>> Cannot push the vacuum
>>
>> In using the dishwasher - cannot carry more than 2 plates
>>
>> Have a yard person come to mow lawn, trim and rake
>>
>> Cannot handle the snow shoveling
>>
>> Laundry - husband does his, I do about 2 loads per week

SHOPPING:
> Used to:
>> Go on all day shopping trips and enjoy it.
>
> Now:
>> Go only at quiet times
>>
>> Take short trips - less than 1 hour
>>
>> Drive until I find a close parking spot
>>
>> Cannot carry packages far - put some into car before continuing
>>
>> Move car to a second spot rather than walk to next store
>>
>> Take breaks - sit down
>>
>> Decide to go home rather than finish my list
>>
>> Have to be careful to stay pleasant
>>
>> Have difficulty when clerks ask too many questions
>>
>> Go with only one idea as a goal

HOBBIES:

    Used to:

        Home decorate - painting, wallpapering, finish
            furniture

        Do complex sewing

        Garden - canning, freezing, preserves

    Now:

        Read, learn computer, art, simple sewing

SOCIAL:

    Used to:

        Be the planner and organizer

        Outgoing personality

    Now:

        Forgotten social engagements

        Had to cancel - too tired

        Cut short the time we stay - worn out the next day

        Need to sit at stand up affairs

        Stressful

        Become quiet and unable to hold up a conversation

PERSONAL CARE:

        Cannot remember what clothes go together

        Have written lists to know what I have

        By the time I dress, I feel too tired to go

        Cannot stand the feel of wool or wear nylon hose

        Do not trust myself in the bath if I'm alone in the
            house

February 1998

With the decrease in working ability, I file for Social Security Disability. It is a very long process.

I am forced to make the decision to follow the advice

"Do less now so you can do more later."

March 1998

I'm sitting on the edge of my bed. A sharp pain starts in my back and radiates through out my upper body. No matter what I do, I cannot ease the pain. I go in to see my family doctor. She is very understanding.

May 1998

I research and find a small, more "stylish" wheelchair. My family doctor writes a prescription for the chair which I hang onto. She also suggests a handicap card for our cars.

My legs have been hurting so bad at night. I elevate them with pillows, so my husband and I look into adjustable beds at the local bed store. We buy two twin adjustable beds and put them side by side, using the same king sheets and blankets. This was such a huge step. It is like "giving up." But the rewards are so great!!! We should have gotten the beds years earlier! I can breathe much easier and my legs are so much better - and my husband stops snoring!!! Our kids lay on them to try them out and think they are really comfortable and not "medical" at all.

We learn a good lesson: do not procrastinate when it comes to getting aids. Relieve all the stress you can.

Spring 1998

I'm sitting on the couch, legs resting; late, late at night. It's the "dark" time when the world outside is still. The time of the night when the energy of the world is shifting, before it renews for a new day. The time of night I find hard to sleep through. Perhaps it is because my body has shut down, freeing my brain to function. I've learned to place a pencil and paper and dictionary in my lap. I'm unsure of what my stuck brain will release tonight.

I close my eyes and tap into the changing energy. Searching for feelings, because thoughts often are stuck. I soon start writing phrases all over the paper in no particular order. Opening the dictionary I begin to search for words that can better describe these feelings. While writing I'm slowly relearning to express myself in words. Working the phrases into order like a puzzle, a new poem emerges, a gentle little twist of a thought at the end and it is finished.

Still dark, the birds start to sing, rejoicing in the new day about to begin. Within an hour all is again quiet as the light steals the darkness. The hustle and bustle will begin as all the birds join in a new song. I can now sleep. My brain has had its freedom; it will now be peaceful.

First thing in the morning, I read my notes. I am intrigued with what is written, unsure if anyone else will think it is worthwhile.

"As one door closes, another will open."

June 1998

I type up a report for my six-month University check-up. The past six months have been hard. I have some improvement with clearer thinking and less hunting for words from the addition of Ginkgo Biloba. The Wisconsin Ginseng, however, had to be limited to a 1/2 capsule because it makes me anxious. Fatigue is a big problem with limited walking or standing. My muscles are tight, and swallowing is a problem unless I use a straw. I also found I was not following through on ideas - I would see the gas gauge was on empty, but not know to stop for gas. I research the Eldepryl and find it is used in higher levels in Europe, so I increase it to find a proper dose. Although the time is still limited in what I can do, I feel better doing what I can.

Even though I have a typed report, I still feel so inadequate in how I am reporting my changes to Dr. Brooks. I ask him to better train me in how to report the changes. When I am in his office my brain is in such a shut down.
Zinc, St. John's Wort, Motrin chewable and CLA (conjugated linoleic acid) to lose weight are recommended to try.
I am to try the Motrin chewable to see if it will not upset my stomach like the other ibuprofens do. Research is finding that it is vital that I find an anti-inflammation drug for the prevention of Alzheimer's disease.

Another neuropsychological exam, MRI and EEG are scheduled. Gene testing is not yet feasible...

Summer 1998

I try the St. John's Wort three different times, at three different levels and two brands. Each time it sends me down in mood and keeps me awake at night. There is an interaction with the Eldepryl. In August the pharmacy gives me the name brand Eldepryl capsules when they run out of the selegiline tablets. I notice that the capsules seem to work more effectively, so I ask for the price difference. It is astronomical! I try crushing the tablets inside of an empty gel capsule to increase the effectiveness. It seems to help.

August 1998

The Social Security Disability Claim is denied.
I feel burdened with the prospect of re-filing. Can't just one thing be a bit easier?

September 1998

It takes me weeks to fill out the new paper work for an appeal, a little every day. It does get sent off.

October 1998

Friends of ours are on the high protein diet. So I pick up the book, *Dr. Atkins' New Diet Revolution.* My husband does well on the diet and loses weight. I, however, do not lose weight; but, I do gain energy and that makes me very happy. Protein is needed to feed the brain; 160 to 240 percent increase in protein with a brain injury. (*Brain Repair* Chapter 9. See Chapter III, page 48)
So my diet becomes much more "brain" nourished.
Thanks to friends...

September 3, 1998

I awake with a start in the middle of the night. I've heard a crash of some sort. I lay in bed for a bit, trying to decide what to do. I know all the doors are locked, yet I feel a presence of some sort. If I were in a movie, I could tell by the music they would play just how scared I should be. I gather my strength and get up to take a look around. Often I think I may have heard something only to assume it was in my dream, so there is probably nothing here.

I peek about the house ending up in the bathroom. There on the floor is the book my husband was reading, and his glasses are in the sink. They have fallen off the counter. It is so strange, I tune into the "presence" I feel still.

My father's older brother, George has been stricken by ALS (Lou Gehrig's disease) and has been on life support for several days. Today is the day his only daughter has been advised to stop the life support. She has asked my father to be with her, and to help in the decision. One of our sisters is driving down with our father.

I have a strong sense of who has come through our house. It is Uncle George accompanied by his brother who died in 1996. (The "Do less now so you can do more later" Uncle.)

They arrived in a whirlwind, making sure I know they are here. In the bathroom window, out through the living room picture window, on to the family farm only blocks from our house. Like young men in a race... and not the 80-somethings they were.

I know what their message is. Our cousin is so torn with the decision on the life support. She wants to hold on so tight to any chance for a miracle. She is all alone now. Her mother died of cancer several years ago.

In the morning I call my sister who is going along and tell her to be sure to tell our cousin of the happenings of that early morning and to assure her that her father is free of his pain and has already traveled on.

I see our cousin several months later and relate it all again. She is still not quite ready. But the next summer we talk again, and then she accepts it. She is relieved to know she did not cause his death to come too early.

September 18, 1998

Ninety-something instead of fifty.

Another birthday – spaced 365 days apart – one should hardly notice the change. Set in the middle of four changing seasons disguised as a routine event. Today maybe a little change, not really enough to worry about. An every day occurrence. Maybe a little less mobile, or a little slower, a little more fatigue, a longer nap – changes that take only a slight adjustment. Natural aging, 40 more years, 14600 days, 160 seasons, ½ of an adult lifetime. But condense all that change into a couple of years and it is like day and night.

A lot of the mysterious quirks of the aged now become clear. Ever wonder why the little aged lady up the street always seems to be wearing the same clothes. Doesn't her family ever buy her anything new? My mother used to comment that no matter how many nice outfits my grandmother had, she always was wearing only one or two.

"It takes too much energy!"

I loved to dress! Seasons change, latest designs, mix and match – I did it all. Never would catch me with the same outfit on twice in one week – much less two days in a row. And I'd never change that – it was a part of who I am, my personality. It took a bit of energy – but it was important.

This changed like day and night. No longer do I recognize what matches, or know what fits. Did I wear this yesterday? No time to change. Oh well...

Cooking 101. Is the first cut on an onion horizontal or vertical to keep it from falling apart? How many cakes and meals with missing ingredients?
Relearn...

October 1998
There are four of us sharing a small table in a cozy restaurant. We also share birthday months, so twice a year, spring and fall, we plan our evening out. There has never been a lack of conversation, often we find the evening over too fast. Laughter and stories filling the time.
But not this year.
I cannot find my thoughts.
I cannot understand the stories.
I cannot remember their children's names.
I cannot answer the questions.
It seems so much easier to sit quietly.
Dinner is over early...
I do not want to lose our friends, too.
If only my second grade teacher could see me now. It is hard to believe I am the same girl that had to have scotch tape put across her mouth to keep from talking in school.

The tremors in my hands are making typing on the computer almost impossible. aaaaaaa's all in a row or ;;;;;;;;;; The motor/muscle doctor explains that sometimes it is harder to do a very delicate task than a heavy one. We look into a voice activated computer program.

November 1998
The MRI, EEG, and Neuropsychological examination are on back-to-back appointments. We arrive early in the morning for the neuropsychological testing, only to be told the scheduled doctor is out of the office and the testing will be with his associate.

The whole reason for coming back down to the University is so the testing would be given by the same person, so the comparison would be accurate. Why didn't they have the courtesy to call and let me make the choice as to who I was seeing? I reschedule.

November 29th
Our future daughter-in-law is enrolled in a school of massage therapy. One of her instructors who has studied herbs gives her information on the herb, Gotu Kola.
She brings me a bottle to try.

Upon taking it, I have an overwhelming feeling of "knowing what I have to do." For someone whose thinking process has been lost for years, this is unbelievable!
Not that a "feeling" is the same as the actual "knowing" - at least it is a step in the right direction.

The local health store owner said that college students would take Gotu Kola before exams in order to perform better. It also helps to make the connection between mind and body.

Gotu Kola   Gotu Kola (Hydrocotyle asiatica)

AKA: Indian Pennywort

Contains asiatic acid, asiaticoside, and madecassic acid.

Used in India for centuries.

Gotu Kola is a nervine, stimulating the central nervous
system, and has an energizing effect on the cells of
the brain.

Enhances memory and mental processing, especially
recall of information.

Aids in circulatory problems in lower limbs including
water retention in ankles, swollen feet, and
varicose veins.

Gotu Kola increases brain circulation improving
depression, poor appetite, and fatigue. It has a
calming effect which aids in stress reduction, and
sleep disorders.

By aiding in the building of collagen, Gotu Kola
stimulates the healing of wounds, skin grafts, and
surgical incisions. Topically applied, it also helps
with eczema, skin problems and foot fungus.

Promotes healthy liver, heart, brain, nerves, urinary tract,
circulation, skin, blood, reproductive organs,
digestive organs, ears, hair, spleen, throat, thyroid,
and tonsils.

Nutritionally rich in vitamins and minerals.

(Also see Chapter X, page 185, for new discoveries.)

dreams...

Fall 1998
I am walking along. The road gradually
changes from smooth to rough
with more and more rocks and boulders,
ups and downs. I continue on,
unable to go back.
I am walking and going downhill – it
is rougher and rougher.
At the bottom is a crevice.
I look around seeing only this crevice
extending to my left and right.
The hill behind is too steep to climb.
Across the crevice the land is flatter, yet still
bumpy, still unknown.
I gather all my strength to jump the crevice –
and achieve! I walk a few steps and
a gentle man comes up.
"Turn to the left, you are almost through this,"
he says.
I climb over some more boulders.
The rocks get smaller.
And there are the green fields
with colorful flowers.

dreams...

December 1998
I'm driving this truck type vehicle
that belongs to Wade. I'm not strong
enough to work the brakes right.
I go off the road and down a hill,
still somewhat in control. At the bottom
of the hill (after many bumps) is a gully.
An old man is walking along and he says,
"I like to go this way, don't you?" We turn left.
I reply, "But it has so many bumps, logs,
and holes." We continue on.
I lift the vehicle over the logs with strength
I never knew I had, and make the turns
and find a way. He is walking alongside.
In a bit he replies, "Yes, but look where
we are now – it is so pretty and natural."
We came out of the gully onto a smooth
and natural field with a small incline, but
without danger.
Sun shinning... Peaceful...

December 1998

Another University appointment. The results of the neuro-psychological testing show some decline, but not enough to diagnose anything. Again it is strongly suggested that depression is the key to this illness. One of the problems with having repeated neuropsychological testing is that the questions are always the same and you get to learn the answers, thus using long-term learned memory instead of short-term. Not once in the report was it noted that perhaps the medications were helping, nor was it noted that the tests I failed were administered last when my 4-hour working window was over and actually give a clearer picture of what is happening. I ask if a truer picture would be obtained if I were off the medications.

Dr. Brooks, however, has other thoughts... The fact that the neuropsychological exam has stayed relatively the same posses another question. Is the stability there because there actually has not been any change (a non-progressive syndrome) or because the regimen I am on has actually prevented it from progressing? The MRI does show more lesions giving possibility to an atypical multiple sclerosis or some variant of a small vessel ischemic disease.
Again, no firm answers.
Because of his peaked interest in the herbs, Dr. Brooks has purchased the first available *Physicians Desk Reference for Herbs*. He states that most drugs were originally derived from herbs. So if they don't have a drug to cure this, then it is good to go back to the herbs. He is the only one on his floor to use this guide. We are happy that he is supportive.

Life's Extension

My Child
Oohs and Aahs
Wiggles Delight
Adults Wonder

Effortless Reaching
Boundless Stretching
Snuggly Shaped

Articulated Prattle
Mimicking Babble
Spontaneously Changing

Heartfelt Love
Birthright Trust
Sleepless Sentries

Eyes Explore
Smiles Galore
Mouthful Connexions

Soulful Beauty
Earth's Wisdom
Heavenly Sent

1999

It is early spring and our daughter is pregnant with their first child, expecting in July. They live in Washington, D.C. and I want to go and stay to help them out. There is a special on the air fare so I talk with her on the phone and ask when she wants me there. Not before or for the delivery, but to be there when she comes home are their wishes. How can I purchase my airline ticket now? I take out a calendar and look at the month of July. One date is glowing brightly - July 26th. I tell them I'll arrive on July 27th. They don't have any better ideas so we leave it at that.

A basic day now consists of getting up between 8 and 9 am. Breakfast, dress, and to get organized takes 2 to 3 hours. Sometimes I need to lay back down. I am able to work on one project a day for about 2 - 3 hours. I have a "shut down" of weakness with pain in my legs, back, and arms. Thinking becomes very unclear.

My creative self is very strong and I find myself doing more and more art-type projects. I use my instincts instead of my brain for a lot of skills. My interest in TV is very short and I like quiet - which I could never stand before. I also continue to push to read.

Writing at night is still an obsession. Although I often do not recognize the notes later as mine. They sound pretty good so I'll continue to compile them.

July 1999
Social Security Disability is approved.

With the success of the Gotu Kola, I look for other herbs that may be beneficial and make a difference in my life. I search through listings and descriptions to find herbs that may address my needs.

What I am primarily looking for is an herb to help with the overwhelming sense of fatigue. The American ginseng that I tried is a bit too stimulating for me. It is as if I don't have the strength for the type of energy it produces. Ginseng may be better later on, if I can build up my strength first.

I narrow my search for herbs that help with fatigue. I also look to digestion, as perhaps the foods I eat are not being assimilated properly. I find several.

One is Schizandra fruit, a complementary herb with Gotu Kola. I love fruit, and the name of the herb sounds like our daughter's name, Casandra. I trust in the coincidence and follow my instincts, it is all I have left... I add in Schizandra fruit capsules, starting at one and increasing to three times a day.

Schizandra   (Shisandra chinensis)

Complementary with Gotu Kola.

As an aid in digestion of fat into fatty acids and glycerol, Schizandra will help:

        * improve brain efficiency

        * aid in memory

        * work as an anti-depressant

Schizandra supports sugar levels thereby:

        * fights fatigue

        * improves stamina

        * builds strength

        * increases work capacity

        * aids in preventing stress

        * increases energy

Schizandra supports the kidneys, lung, heart, pancreas,
        intestines, liver, brain, nerves, and muscles.

It is high in vitamins C and E.

It aids in balancing of all body systems.

An anti-oxidant.

Our grandson, Max is born July 26th.......
I arrive on July 27th... happy and relieved that I was able to handle the flight... and... the timing is perfect! I am spending a month with them to help out, and perhaps to give my husband a bit of a respite. It is great for me because after losing my job and all that I had learned in 50 years of life – including how to cook – I find I can still hold a baby!

Dignity is not "the something" anyone else can take from you, but it is "the something" you can take from yourself. It is a self-perception. My daughter allowed me to be a useful grandmother, my Dignity.

Babies' lives move slowly – it takes an hour or more to eat, an hour to look around and learn, and an hour of rest. If you follow that schedule – it is very nourishing for any body... This tiny baby, Max, is showing me the way. My brain is damaged – but it is repairable. A theory just recently proven by science. So, if I do as Max does, I will be giving my body a chance to heal.
"Do less now, so you can do more later," I understand!

I just realized another important fact. Along with losing – and this is extremely hard to admit to --- Try again --- Memories... The channels to my memories are broken. It is like an earthquake has come and heaved up all the paved roads. Now, there is still the land where the memories sit, but the neat little roads are gone. So to get to these memories is no longer easy. I often see them sitting there, but I have to find a new way and make a new path.

Sometimes that path is not as strong as the roads and it gets blown away again.
So I again lose my way there.

How does Max help with this?
It's now Christmas time and Max is 7 months old and still living in Washington, D.C., we live in Wisconsin. I have been lucky to see him about once every 4 to 5 weeks for a week at a time. We are very close.

Each time it takes a bit before he knows who I am. And then it is OK with him – he'll have a smile, or we'll play our little games. This time he has it all figured out. It took a bit and then he shows me he knows. We are together on the couch when he just grabs hold tight and gives me hundreds of slobbery kisses. He buries his head in my chest and tummy, just like how we always held him to burp. He holds on tight. We squeal in delight together and hug ever so tight. Later as I am giving him an early morning bottle, after his burp, he wiggles until he gets his now 29" long frame of a body all pulled up and tucked in. He falls asleep on my chest like a little ball... how he used to in the first months of his life. We enjoy the closeness and I hold him tightly – and then in 15 minutes or so he stretches back out "like a big boy" to let me know it is fun to go back and visit, but "I'm bigger now."

So how does this help me?
I must have patience and the faith of a child.
Try again, it will come.

Connections
I've read several theories about mind/body and
mind/body/heart connections. That not all our
"memories" are stored in the brain, so if we feel a
soft blanket we may remember a baby.
The heart holds its own neuro center so thinking with
the heart is like this:
A brain sees a cure, a heart sees healing.

Perhaps this helps explain how I have so many
"emotional memories" even though I can not seem
to remember exact events.
If I can no longer use my "brain" then I will use my
heart. If I cannot figure it out mathematically, then
I'll do it by feel or artistically.

"Learn to Listen with Your Heart"

My mother-in-law and I are working on a baby quilt.
I struggle and struggle to measure and balance the
squares using a ruler. What should have been so
easy - I started sewing at the age of nine - seems so
impossible.

So I set the ruler down, look at the squares, and let
my hands and the artistic side of my brain work.
The quilt turns out wonderfully!

Hannah's Heirs - What an excellent book to bring a personal insight into the hereditary factor and history of early onset Alzheimer's Disease. Knowing that there are so many dedicated researchers all over the world is a great comfort. Maybe our family fits into one of these lines.

Hannah's Heirs   The Quest for the Genetic Origins of Alzheimer's Disease   by Daniel A Pollen, M.D., Professor of Neurology and Physiology, Un. of Mass. Medical Center   1993, 1996 update
Printed with permission from Oxford University Press,
198 Madison Ave, NY

A story of research on pedigree families across the world all with early-onset Alzheimer's but with varying pathological findings. And the search for the mutated genes causing this disease.

First studied and named for:

1907 Alois Alzheimer -

Aphasia – an inability to express speech or comprehend language. "Spoke without intonation." In her conversation, she often used confused phrases, single paraphasic expressions (milk-jug instead of cup), some times she would stop talking completely. She evidently did not understand many questions.

Amnesia – an unrelenting impairment of memory

Apraxia – inability to carry out a previously
learned skilled action in the absence of a
motor weakness or a sensory abnormality.

Agnosia – the inability to recognize or identify a
familiar object

Apathetic – without interest

In the end, confined to bed, in a fetal position,
incontinent.

Amyloid plaques and neurofibrillary tangles.

1   Hannah's Heirs

A family linked to Hannah & Shlomo. Lithuania

Hannah born 1844 died at age of 50, 1894

Gave birth to 9 children between 1869 and 1888

All the children helped with her care, down to
assisting with combing her hair, recent
memory and her personal care.

Jewish oppression, famine, at some point moved to
Ekaterinoslave.

Heirs living in USA

Classic symptoms for familial Alzheimer's
Onset age between 42-54
Memory loss
Personal care needed

ALS (amyotophic lateral scerosis) also in family

Familial Hyperlipidemia also in family (heart)
CHROMOSOME 14 (6.99)

2 Italian Pedigree - Robert Feldman\ Chief Neurology at Boston University and Ronald Polinsky\ National Institute of Health

A scientific study started in 1960's with Italian kindred in **France, Italy, and USA**

Collaborators:Bruni, Foncin, Supino-Viterbo, Salmon

4000 known descendants, 60 known cases, 5 living in 1988, all descended from a common ancestor - a woman called Vittoria, born in 1715 in mountain village in the province of Calabria at the southern tip of Italy

Often seizures or brain wave (EEG) abnormalities suggestive of a seizure disorder occurring very early in the course of the disease

Mental deterioration

Aphasia

In later phases, their faces remained immobile, their limbs were held as if in a "plastic rigidity," and their body postures, even while lying in bed, were contorted, with their upper and lower limbs flexed in an exaggerated manner toward their bodies.

Signs of forgetfulness appeared extremely early, between ages of 30 and 40 with 8 of the 13 cases (over 4 generations) starting in their 30's and 2 cases at age 31 and 32.

Temporal lobes had numerous senile plaques,

neurofibrillary tangles, and granulovacuolar changes fitting the diagnostic criteria for Alzheimer's. And neurofibrillary tangles were found in parts of the basal ganglia, such as the claustrum, putamen, and globus pallidus, where the pathology might explain the disorders of movement and posture, and in the dentate nucleus of the cerebellum, where the pathology might explain the spontaneous jerky contractions of individual muscle groups that were also very frequent in affected members.

Also noted was degeneration of the anterior horn cells or "motor neurons" in the spinal cord, which was presumed to have led to the atrophy of some of the muscle groups.

CHROMOSOME 14   (5.38)   chromosome 21 (2.56)

3   **Dutch Belgium Family -Christine Van Broeckhoven**

Familial Alzheimer's disease with predominant vascular involvement.

Four families living in the Netherlands with a hereditary condition cerebral amyloid angiopathy. Amyloid accumulates in the walls of cerebral blood vessels and leads to brain hemorrhages in adults in their fifth and sixth decades of life.

Dementia shows up in later stages, if survived

A mutation at position 22 – cytosine (C) for guanine (G) in the APP gene 21

CHROMOSOME 14

4   **British Canadian   Linda Nee, Ronald Polinsky, and Peter Hyslop**

Husband of a woman born in Northumberland, England, in 1763, who died young, was presumed to be the carrier.

The mother and a number of children immigrated to New Brunswick, Canada in 1837.

Numerous descendents developed dementia in midlife.

By the seventh generation in 1960s and 1970s were seeing descendants in their early or mid-fifties affected.

Classic symptoms of familial Alzheimer's

Identical to Hannah's family

CHROMOSOME 14 (3.99)

5   **English Family   John Hardy / St. Mary's Hospital Medical School, London**

Familial Alzheimer's disease

Deposition of amyloid in the fine cerebral blood vessels

Markedly increased incidence of thyroid disease in the affected members

A mutation in exon 17 – cytosine (C) in place of thymine (T)

6   **Volga Germans**   **Gerard Schellenberg/ Seattle**
Thomas Bird

American descendants of a small group of settlers
whose ancestors had emigrated from two
adjacent villages in the Southern Volga
region of Russia.

In 1762 Catherine Empress of Russia, herself of
German birth, invited settlers from Western
Europe to settle and farm the open plains
south along the river Volga to curtail the
series of invasions by marauding tribes from
Central Asia.

Life in Germany had been oppressive. Not much
better in Russia. Formed towns of Frank
and Walter. WWI many Volga Germans
headed for U.S.

Settled in Midwestern states of Dakotas, Kansas,
Nebraska, Colorado, and West Coast. By
1980's there were some 300,000 American
descendants of Volga Germans.

Unusual 15 year spread in mean onset of
Alzheimer's – age mid 40's through 63.

CHROMOSOME 1   presenilin 2

(Functional significance of the chromosome 1 and 14
mutations are apt to be the same as the amino acid
sequence are so similar)

A map of our ancestors' homelands.

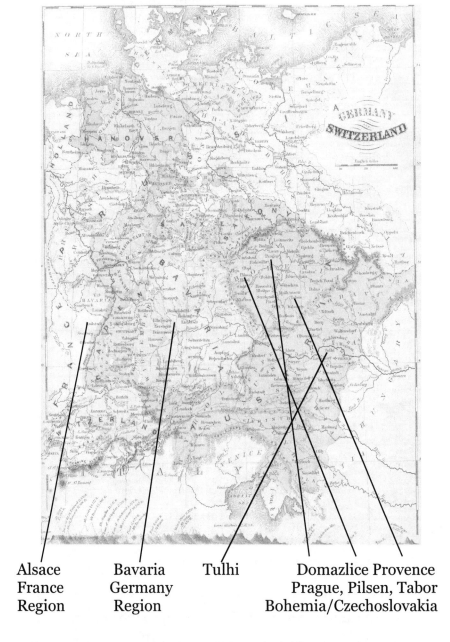

Alsace Bavaria Tulhi Domazlice Provence
France Germany   Prague, Pilsen, Tabor
Region Region   Bohemia/Czechoslovakia

Our mother's sister, Mary Louise, has spent a great deal of
her life researching our heritage, back to the 1800's.
This is a map of the regions where they lived.

November 1999

I have found my intelligence tests taken in high school.

I now have the proof of who I was. I am amazed, they are all pegged in the 95-100 percentile range...

And here I am - or what is left, barely functioning at average - some in the demented... but then they don't see that I feel a loss - because I am still able to find ...

Average!

I have lost 50% of who I am - but because I don't fall below a particular mark, I am not yet "diseased"!

Well, they are wrong!

I have tried to always tell you - what "they" say is not set in gold! It is what your instincts tell you. Again I have proof. Why don't "they" just listen to those who are experiencing it? It's not really important. It is ME who matters and what I know. But then what about all the "others" who are struggling with me? I am not the only one in this situation. I'm the lucky one who can still see what is happening and try to yell and scream and have "them" listen and help us "others."

Before it IS too late.

December 1999

It is Christmas time. My husband is very frustrated because
he says, for once, he has an excellent gift idea but is having
trouble finding what he wants.

Christmas comes. We open our gifts. He hands me two
small boxes. Inside the first I find a beautiful rose pendent.
The second holds a ring with a beautiful rose shaped from
Black Hill's gold. He tells me the roses are so that I think
often of my mother, Buelah Rose.

He may never realize how important that simple gesture
was. Or how much it means to me. How he gave me
strength when I was doubting myself. He is affirming his
support in my research. He is standing by my side, when it
would be so much easier to turn away.

I talk of my intuitions, my feelings of how close my mother
is, her guidance; and he does not think I am crazy! He is
offering me support, encouragement, and
his healing love...

Chapter VIII

Love is...

Love is...
A Reassuring Nod
A Gentle Touch in Passing
Close Held Hands
Caressing Moments
All Encompassing Eyes
Commingled Minds

Love is filled with...
Trusting Souls
Shared Courage
Respectful Views
Honored Identity
Generous Sharing
Understood Limits
Heartfelt Pain

Love is to be...
Held in Wonder
Fulfilled in Joy
Grown in Harmony
Faithfully Nurtured
Thereby...
Lasting

Spring 2000

"Today is better"

I awoke this morning to find some more of "The Me Inside." It keeps coming back in such small steps. But then that must be the way it has to be because that is how it was lost – little steps at a time.

dreams.....

In the dream I am at a social event and a man comes up to me and starts talking as if he knows who I am – wanting to know what has happened in my life. We talk a bit and I am telling him, yet in such a positive light no longer saying "I am disabled." But saying, "I have been struggling with a neuro-logical problem." We are interrupted by another girl who places herself next to him. A dance starts and they drift away, but as everyone turns to the music he steps next to me and takes my hand. At the touch of his hand I remember all of 1967 – I know places, peoples' faces, and names – all of which I have been struggling to remember for so many years!

He was my boss at the time. It was a good job, working in bookkeeping/accounting. I awake, and for the next hour let my memories flow – back to 8th grade. Filling in some of the black. Not empty, but black. If it were empty then you don't know it was once there – if it is black (or white) then you know of it, but can't find it. Is that so important? It makes me fear the fact that I will bump into those in the black and not be able to respond to them. They know all that I can no longer find.

How embarrassing!

It happens so often – I get this genuine smile from someone and I am lost – stumbling past. Or I see a face, want to go up and say "Hi," but I am not sure enough to do it – so I put my head down and hope they don't see me.

It is so complicated. Everything - everything has to be in balance. I have to have done enough in a day to stimulate – but not overload; I have had to eat enough protein for energy balanced with enough carbohydrates so I can sleep. I have to have enough medication to relieve the tremors, inflammation, and balance the blood pressure and lastly the right nutritional mix to achieve.

When I get it perfect then I get closer.
Closer to not just healing, but to curing.

Fall 2000
"I no longer feel sick. I feel handicapped, but not sick.."

dreams...

> I am at a reunion of sorts. I can recognize others from prior years, we are familiar enough to have been family – at first I thought it was a convention. There are many rooms and each person has a different responsibility in their own room. Yet you go freely to visit in all the rooms. My husband knows I'm there – he and our son.

He says, "It's hard to find the way there, I'm not sure I can tell you. But once you're there, the way back is easy."
I meet up with a young lady who has had brain cancer but has fought it off several times. We mingle. I'm outside for a moment. The outside is like our homestead, driveway and house. I roll off the driveway into the orchard and watch as my grandmother (my father's mother) is taken away. She has died.

I'm back inside the building and come upon a group of children. It is my job to set up microscopes and show them these really interesting slides that were just found after being lost for a long time. I look at the slides in my hand and realize how familiar and interesting they are. We have trouble setting up the microscopes because the plug in the wall is hard to reach. The kids say, "Let's go up to the next floor – it is new and has desks with plugs made for these microscopes." I say "No, this is my floor and we'll make do," (the easiest floor is not always the best.) I rearrange the tables and chairs and it works, although not in a perfect order. But when they look at the slides they no longer care that this set-up is more difficult.

I leave them and come upon a group of mixed ages. The young lady who had the brain cancer is there. She has a baby and husband at home. I can talk with her in a language we both understand, but not everyone else can. She gets word that her child at home has inherited her brain cancer and has died.

There is a "child" although very wise and knowing, who walks by. She is dressed in blue and is very powerful. Deep eyes. I walk into another room with others. We hear a rumble and small noise from the previous room. The lady who had the brain cancer has died.

The "child" in blue comes to me. I know who she is. She comes when you are to die. I am not afraid. I am lying down, warm with a blanket. She touches me gently. I feel her touch against my skin; it is soft and warm. My whole body shakes as if to separate a part of me - when the separation is complete I will have "died" - but actually only have left behind my body and traveled on.

The "shaking" awakens me. I am now aware of what is happening. I hear my husband's breathing next to me and think of my family. I am at peace.

I am very cold, yet under all these blankets, I should be warm. I breathe deeply and find I am fully here. When you miss a death "they" have to heal another part of you - to make life a bit easier. Because it means you have something more to accomplish and "they" have to make it a bit easier - it's a trade. Feels good.

2000

The medications have helped, but they are so "short lived" - hours instead of full days. I am choosing one task per day not lasting more than 2 to 3 hours.

I research the herbs looking for an herb that will help with my stamina and address the Parkinsonian symptoms. I seek herbs that will complement, not interfere with my medications. If it is also good for the brain, then that will be a bonus.

My choices are: Broad Bean, Cayenne, Damiana, Passion Flower, Pau d' Arco and Wood Betony. I chose to try Damiana.

Damiana   (Turnera aphrodisiaca)

Damiana has long been known as a strengthener of male and female reproductive organs. Aiding in infertility (men and women), menopause, and hot flashes.

Lesser known is that Damiana is a central nervous system stimulant. Aiding in loss of power to limbs, and stimulating the muscles of the intestinal tract.

Damiana helps with:

* dizziness
* vertigo
* exhaustion
* energy
* nervousness
* Emphysema
* acne
* fungus and Athlete's foot

Damiana will aid in Parkinson's Disease.

Damiana supports the reproductive organs, brain, nerves, kidneys, lungs and skin.

May 2000

A yearly check-up at the University shows a stability. The addition of the herb Damiana has helped to overcome some of the exhaustion and helps with my walking and lifting. It is also a good hormone balancer and nervine (strengthens functional activity of the nervous system.) Because I am lousy at cooking fish I have also added salmon oil for Omega 3's.

I relate the dreams I have recorded. Dr. Brooks states that dreams are a big way to heal and it is important that they are positive. Psyche healing sometimes occurs before physical healing.

When we first had appointments at the University with our mother it was the norm to bring only the patient into the room. Our family pretty much changed that because she was unable to communicate well. It was soon known that when we arrived the nurses would have to bring in extra chairs for our family.

Being a research hospital/clinic often there has to be "proof" or some way to document symptoms. Alzheimer's is extremely difficult because so far the only way to be sure of the diagnosis is by dissecting the brain. Dr. Brooks told us today he has learned over the years to listen to his patients and he is now passing that knowledge onto his son, who is in medical school, so that his son will benefit.

It is very meaningful to our family to have a doctor who is not limited and will grow with experience along with us.

A letter to my family:

Family news   Fall 2000

It has been awhile since you have heard from our family.
I'd like to take the time to give you some information on the
research I have been doing on Alzheimer's Disease. I choose
this time because I believe I have enough information to make
a difference.

Recap: Buelah's neuropathologic diagnose was a posterior
dementia due to a combination of Alzheimer's Disease with
amyloid angiopathy. In addition there was granulovacuolar
degeneration and PAS plaques. The amyloid angiopathy is a
hereditary form of Alzheimer's. There were unique features
of lacunar changes in the basal ganglia and cribriform changes
in the cerebral white matter, and an involvement of the
substantia nigra and locus caeruleus.

Lots of big words!

Basically it says that there were a lot more physical problems
along with the usual mental problems associated with basic
Alzheimer's. Also this type is generally seen at an earlier onset - with a lot of the physical problems expressed first sometimes causing early death. The hereditary factor is 50%. I
have been going to the University of Madison Clinic since
1990. And similar to Mama's, they cannot tell us exactly what
is going on. But, there is a form of Alzheimer's that includes
Parkinsonian like symptoms (one of the more than 30 types
now found). And this is the closest.

I can explain it like an earthquake has rumbled through my brain, heaving up all the roads to my memories and thoughts. Taking me forward in life until I felt like I was 90 years old. To get to the memories or even to find them was a monumental task. There have been times when I have been so bad that I could not walk up a few steps, or get up off a chair without help, or was so moody my own children were afraid of me, or that I had to have others do my job because I couldn't remember how, or shook so bad I would not eat soup, or was so weak I could not lift a bottle of milk. So you see the brain affects every aspect of the body - or sometimes only a small part.

What I want to tell you today is that we have been able to manage most of these problems and I have been stable for the second year in a row! I am determined to rebuild those roads. Like other illnesses there is no one magic pill - but a whole "cocktail." **Each person will be unique**.

MOST IMPORTANT - a lot can be done for prevention and strengthening of your system! You do not have to go where I am. Ginkgo Biloba, vitamin E, and others are already proven to delay Alzheimer's by 5 years. High B vitamins with Folic Acid is a brain regenerator. The earlier the better. Thus my letter to each of you.

First off - always remember "When one door closes - another will open." I was terrified - there was no way I wanted to be looking down the throat of this beast that brings so much pain and separation. The idea of losing who I am, the change in going from being depended upon to dependent is very hard on a family. But I have found some new parts of me, in having to slow down it has been good to explore what else I am capable of. Also, every minute of every day is now important to me and is shared with my family and friends. A lot of people don't get to feel that.

There are four aspects in what is working for me:

1 Nutrition - A balanced diet for me – I threw those food charts out the window! I found I was starving myself trying to eat too low fat. A high protein diet and at this point not worry about fat - low on refined, simple carbohydrates - add in the Omega3 oils with salmon - include vitamins, minerals, and herbs. Organic foods, if possible, and watch for heavy metals. Our neurologist in Madison has the first available book for physicians on herbs - he states most medicines were formulated from herbs.

2 Mind and Body Exercise - Right now mostly mind exercises. Relearning to read, sew, cook, etc. Physical exercise is limited to non-repetitive movements.

3 Stress Management - A realization that even the smallest things like the environment can hold stress for me. I didn't realize just how much physical stress the tremors alone were causing. Taking time to find the "Bliss." In finally getting up enough nerve to tell my Madison doctor that not only are the herbs helping, but that I am also reading on Eastern ideas of healing, he simply stated that healing has to occur in the psyche first.

4 Pharmacology - Good old pills

Following is a list of medicines and supplements I am taking:

Amantadine	to stop the Parkinson-like tremors. Mine has to be the yellow brand as I am allergic to the red ones (Mama was also)
Eldepryl	to put the connection back between my brain and my body. With this I can walk, write, talk, etc. This is a Parkinson drug, but taken early on it, also, holds promise in slowing Alzheimer's.
Atenolol	blood pressure
Zincate	low zinc is prevalent in this disease
Multi Vitamin	3 times per day. This was the first addition to my diet. I found that when I took it I felt better for a short time. (9 years ago) And with trial I have found I still need this level.
Ginkgo Biloba	words come out of my head - and they are even right! Most of the time - when I take this. Otherwise I have trouble finding the right word or some times some pretty "dicey" words pop up. It increases the blood flow to the brain bringing oxygen and nutrition.
WI Ginseng	this helps the body, but I have to be very careful because it is often too strong
Vitamin E	anti-oxidant. A preventative and aids in healing.
Aspirin	one baby, as a preventative
Advil	as a preventative
Omega 3	nutrition basic

Gotu Kola	this is in the ginseng family, but a little milder. It helps with that connection between my brain and my body. It is also a mild "feel good" herb. I was unable to tolerate St. John's Wort. This also helps with memory and learning. I feel this is as important as the Ginkgo Biloba.
Schizandra	aids in the digestion of fat to fatty acids and glycerol. Supports sugar levels, boosts stamina, moistens dry and irritated tissues. For me it opened my air passages so I could breathe better and improved swallowing.
CoQ10 /Lecithin	good for the heart and circulation.
Damiana	helps overcome exhaustion and helps to restore the loss of power in my limbs. A hormone balancer as all functions of the body are regulated by hormones and a nervine.

This may seem like a lot to take, but then I was pretty bad, and a lot of it is nutritional. I also mix the herbs rather than take a full dose of one as they work better in combination. A few words on the foods I eat. I have forgotten about the word "fat" and have concentrated on the protein. If I go with the book on diet and your blood type, my blood type is O and I am a meat eater! When blood sugar drops, cortisol is released, which makes me nervous, jittery, and anxious. Cortisol is the "fear and flight" hormone. My system doesn't shut it off once started, and I'll be "up" for days after any hard stress. Cortisol, when unchecked, damages the brain. I also found I may have a sugar sensitivity, so I have cut way back on that. Along with that are the carbohydrates - wheat seems to be a big problem. A wheat sensitivity can cause brain swelling. And the whole concept of the Vitamin E, Advil and Aspirin is to reduce inflammation of the brain. Diet appears to be one of the main links to the weakness in the brain. The simple carbohydrates we eat increase the production of insulin, which increase the production of cholesterol, and factors into Type II Diabetes. I am also trying to eat organic foods most often. The brain needs specific proteins to function - and this links back to the foods we eat and how they are digested. Did you know that Alzheimer's first appeared in cultures after there were years of famine?

I have been looking for the link among the diseases we have seen in Mama's family. How do heart disease, stroke, diabetes, goiter, and Alzheimer's relate? Where do depression, learning problems and alcohol intolerance fit in? It appears it may be hyperinsulinemia (excess insulin) and insulin resistance. And that comes down to the foods we eat and how our systems digest them. I remember Mama telling us that food was scarce during their early years and that they would have popcorn for breakfast because there was nothing else. What we don't know is what comes first, the brain damage or the digestion/absorption problems.

"Do less now, so you can do more later." These were the words of advice from our uncle upon his deathbed. I found this to be the hardest – with our "go, go, go, do, do, do" ancestry. So the last piece to put together is "Bliss." The body cannot repair unless it is given the time to do so. And this means finding your own way of "closing down and just feeling good." I especially like holding my sleeping grandson. Babies are so snuggly (note I said "sleeping grandson") and you can just feel the love circling around. Each time we spend time together, I come home stronger. Find nature and its strengths. Wherever it is for you.

It is hard to tell you if we have found all the pieces to the puzzle when we don't know how many there are - but I can say I think it is getting very close. Each new piece makes such a difference.

How did I find this information? I am a very "have to know" person. After the years of not knowing with Mama I was driven to find out. One of the biggest breakthroughs came when my son and his fiancée had driven me to Madison. We shopped on State Street as a treat. Looking around at shelves and shelves of books in this unique store I picked out a book and paged through. The information was fascinating and extremely helpful. Whenever I was ready for more information, I'd walk through a book store and was never let down. I've learned to trust my instincts and listen to the coincidences of life. I will follow with a list of the books I have used for reference. I don't want to overdo this information. I hope this information will help to end the hereditary link. It has given me closure to be able to pass this information on to you with confidence that it is complete enough to make a difference and that I am able to back it up with medical validity and not just "my instincts." I must be near to completing the puzzle as I am no longer "obsessed."

Lots of love.

BOOKS FOR HOPE

THE AMAZING BRAIN   (copyright) 1984
   Robert Ornstein & Richard F. Thompson
   Houghton Mifflin Co. Publisher
A visual view of the brain anatomy, mechanisms, and process.
A 1984 edition - already outdated but good for basics.

HOSTAGE BRAIN   1994
   Bruce McEwen & Harold M. Schmeck, Jr.
   Rockefeller University Press
A look into how the brain works and what goes wrong when it
is injured or diseased.

BRAIN REPAIR   1995
   Donald G. Stein, Simon Brailowsky, Bruno Will
   Oxford University Press, New York
A study into the theory of neuroplasticity which stresses that
cells throughout the brain can not only regenerate, but can
adapt their function to assume critical roles once performed by
damaged tissue. Cells called Glial cells play an essential role in
the growth and survival of nerve cells. Glia does a number of
good things to help the brain repair itself. Enhancement of
Glia cells is achieved through pharmacology, nutrition and
most important mental exercises. It also talks about the
negative effects of stress - be it due to physical limitations,
emotions, or environment. This book gave me hope that I may
be able to stay ahead of the progressive decline. The
question was, "How?"

HANNAH'S HEIRS   1996

The Quest for the Genetic Origins of Alzheimer's Disease

Daniel A. Pollen, MD   Oxford University Press, NY

Here is a compilation of the genetic tree for Alzheimer's. Included is the study of seven main family pedigrees suffering from forms of Alzheimer's back to the 1800's in Italy, France, Lithuania, Germany, Canada, and USA. These families also had a higher incidence of thyroid, ALS (Lou Gehrig's disease), hyperlipidemia heart disease, and Down's Syndrome. Age of onset varied by family, some as early as 30 years old. Symptoms varied from the typical Alzheimer's to include seizures, involvement of the basil ganglia and horn cells, or hemorrhage without dementia until late in life if survived. Noted was that all families appeared to have gone through a period of starvation due to famines or wars. This book has strong "Notes" and "Reference" chapters. Aunt Mary Louise's heredity chart was most helpful.

MOLECULES OF EMOTION   1997

Candace B. Pert, Ph.D.

Simon & Schuster Publishing

"Laughter is the best medicine." This book reveals that "emotions" are actually molecules called Peptides. These chemicals play a wide role in regulating practically all life processes. They are part of a chemical system which is made up of neurotransmitters (made in the brain to carry information between one neuron and the next i.e. dopamine, serotonin, etc.) and steroids (sex hormones) and peptides (which link brain-to-body and body-to-brain). Memories are stored not only in the brain, but in a psychosomatic network extending into the body. They are molecules and not, as previously thought, electrical impulses. Also it has been found that the immune system can communicate with the endocrine system, the nervous system and the brain. The peptides integrate this system forming a psycho-immunoendocrine network. By laughing we can release natural endorphins (a peptide) that will give pain relief and a feeling of euphoria. We can start to have control!

BOOKS FOR ACTION!

BRAIN LONGEVITY   1997
   Dharma Singh Khalsa, MD   Warner Books
By incorporating Eastern and Western medicine traditions and the latest research on brain chemistry, this book reveals how nutritional therapy (including diet, natural medicinal tonics, and nutritional supplementation), mind and body exercise, stress management, and pharmacology can slow the aging process and help reverse brain degeneration. This is a very good resource.

PARKINSON'S DISEASE   1993
   Abraham N. Lieberman, MD and Frank L. Williams
                                 Firestone Books
My resource for the Parkinsonian type symptoms that are so
apparent. An educational and practical guide to controlling
these. There is a strong overlap in all neurodegenerative
diseases.

THE HIGHLY SENSITIVE PERSON   1996
   Elaine N Aron, Ph.D.   Broadway Books
Many in our family seem to fit this profile. This book will help
identify if you are a highly sensitive person. Between
15% -20% of the population has a sensitive nervous system
that is stimulated by subtleties in the environment, other
people's moods, strong smells, coarse fabrics, deeply moved by
arts or music, etc. Was school hard - just being there? Here is
information on how to recognize and reduce the stress that
accompanies this sensitivity. How to keep from being over-
stimulated. A stress reducer. And - to match your career to
the wonderful gift you have - you were born to be among the
advisors and thinkers, the spiritual and moral leaders of your
society. "Shy and Sensitive" are not bad attributes.

EAT RIGHT 4 YOUR TYPE   1996
   Dr. Peter J. D'Adamo   Catherine Whitney
   G.P. Putnam's Sons Publishing
A look into how your blood type may effect what you eat. Is
there a connection between blood type (which also goes along
the lines of nationality), food, and disease?

POTATOES NOT PROZAC   ARE YOU SUGAR
SENSITIVE?   1998
   Kathleen DesMaisons, Ph.D.   Fireside Books
How to balance low blood sugar, low levels of Serotonin, and
low levels of beta-endorphin (the natural feel good peptide)
with the foods we eat. Optimal blood sugar brings energy,
focus, good memory, and concentration. Optimal serotonin
levels bring hope, creativity, and optimism. Optimal levels of
beta-endorphin give tolerance to pain, high self-esteem,
compassion and a desire to take personal responsibility. It is a
low sugar, high protein, nutritional way to eat.

DR. ATKINS' NEW DIET REVOLUTION   1997
   Robert C. Atkins, M.D.   Avon Health
An introduction to a high protein, low carbohydrate life style.

BEYOND PROZAC   1996
   Michael J. Norden, M.D.   Regan Books
Covers serotonin deficiency, stress, and "natural prozac."
Includes a good chapter on essential fats. Also includes a
glycemic index of carbohydrates.

PRESCRIPTION FOR NUTRITIONAL HEALING   1997
   James F. Balch, MD and Phyllis A. Balch, CNC
   Avery Publishing Group
This is one of my reference books for the herbs, vitamins,
minerals, and food supplements.

PROTEIN POWER   1998
   Revised PROTEIN POWER LIFEPLAN   2000
   Michael R. Eades, M.D.   Mary Dan Eades, M.D.
                          Warner Books

A much more complete, medical explanation of the high
protein life style. Goes much more in depth between the
relationship of heart disease, diabetes, and brain energy.
Also omega 3 fatty acids, eicosanoids, and arachidonic acid
sensitivity (which can cause chronic fatigue, poor sleep,
brittle hair). Lots of information on cholesterol. A very good
source for diet, including need of complex carbohydrates.

BOOKS FOR THE SPIRIT

CELESTINE PROPHECY   1993
   James Redfield   Warner Books

Drawing on ancient wisdom, a guidebook that helps your
perceptions of why you are where you are in life... and to
direct your steps with a new energy and optimism for
tomorrow. A sharing in ideas of energy, intuition and
coincidences.

SECOND SIGHT   1996
   Judith Orloff, M.D.   Warner Books

An insight into the psychic experiences in everyday life.
How to accept them and not fear them.

QUANTUM HEALING   1990
Exploring the Frontiers of Mind/Body Medicine.
       Deepak Chopra, M.D.   Bantam Publishing
A combination of the current research of Western medicine,
neuroscience, and physics with the insights of India Ayurvedic
theory to show that the human body is controlled by a network
of intelligence grounded in quantum reality. By finding
"bliss" - a time of quiet - the body is able to rebalance and start
to heal. This is a scientific approach to Eastern medicine
(which my analytical mind needed).

THE HEART'S CODE   1999
       Paul Pearsall, Ph.D.   Broadway Books
Through his work as a well-credentialed psychologist
studying heart transplant patients, Dr. Pearsall shows how the
heart thinks, remembers, communicates, helps regulate
immunity, and contains stored information. Explaining the
theory and science behind energy cardiology. The brain says
we are healed when numbers from machines tell us we are
"back in the normal range." The heart says, whether or not we
are cured, that we are healed when we feel whole. When we
have learned to celebrate life rather than just struggle to
prolong it and when we have learned how to be more aware of
the loving energy flowing freely within us again.

By seeing the heart as the center of my life, the changes in
my brain are not so threatening - I can still be me.
And that gives me the power to heal.

                                   Chris

Seeters

My Child
Nighttime Laughter
Unjudging Trust
Secrets locked in Jeweled Boxes

Harmonic Spirits
Shared Minds
Delicate sensitivities Protected

Sassy Communications
Bonded Energies
Trellised paths Fulfilled

Duplicate Smiles
Gathered Hands
Ageless Wonders grown Together

With Love
Sisters

February 2001

With the reduction in my overall body pain, I note that I am now aware of having arm pain and a tightness in my chest upon exertion (which does not seem to take much effort). It may have been going on for some time, but pain is what I have been living with. My family doctor sends me for a treadmill stress test - which I fail.

Both of our mother's brothers died of heart problems when they were in their early sixties, so we have a very real threat. I am told the next step is an arterogram. I really do not want to have this done. I am concerned that the procedure itself will set me back. I contact Dr. Brooks at the University clinic. He personally calls me back after talking with the heart doctor and tells me I will have the procedure.

The arterogram shows no blockage to the heart. I pass. The heart doctor was hoping he could help me with some of the symptoms I have been experiencing. He looks very discouraged. He makes sure that I will be seeing Dr. Brooks soon. I come through the procedure, but there is still a mystery as to why the lack of oxygen in the heart.

My family doctor has also set me up with an appointment at a new local Memory Center that she is very pleased with.

April 2001

My younger sister takes the afternoon off from work to go with me to the appointment at The Memory Center, Affinity Health System, Oshkosh, WI. She is spending so much of her time accompanying family members to our various appointments.

The cognitive testing at the Memory Center is very extensive. They also interview my sister to get an outside perspective of me. I see Dr. Janelle Cooper who asks a lot of background questions. She feels she may have some clues into what is going on. And she is encouraging in that she may have some other ideas. A high definition MRI is ordered along with a repeat neuropsychological assessment. The MRI is to be given at a specific hospital where Dr. Cooper has worked with the technicians to get the best view possible.

May 2001

I am back at the Memory Center for the results of the MRI and testing. The neuropsychological exam has not yet been done because of his busy schedule. I have come alone because of everyone's commitments for the day.

Entering the room along with Dr. Cooper are two other women. I sense all the "clues for a fixable situation" are gone. Dr. Cooper tells me the very specific MRI shows more damage, lesions. It is now very clear there have been scattered small strokes, vascular in type. No other possibility is discussed - how very different - how technology can make the difference. Based on their location they may affect my planning ability. That is not a maybe, because that is just what is happening.

Dr. Cooper is so much more serious as she shakes her head and tries to think of some other answer she can give me without my even asking. One of the women present has been taking notes for me. I think what a nice way to help out. An adult aspirin is added to my medications until I go back to the University clinic. We also discus the importance of the Omega 3's, which I will increase. She stresses the importance of a strong preventative approach for Alzheimer's Disease.

I am introduced to the women, a social worker and an Alzheimer's Association Representative. Both ask if there is anything I need help with. They feel I have been making the adjustment well and I have strong family support. I only need to ask, they will always be there for me.

I now know what path I am on....

Often my research and commitment to finding the answers has been viewed as an "obsession." But I have always felt that I have only a limited time to achieve. At some point, I am not going to be able to communicate my feelings. I am not going to be able to tell you what is better, what is worse.

I will not give up unless I can no longer think - or no longer tell you what I thought, which might come first.

My older sister lives in the same city as the University.
In November 1999, she experienced a visual aura. She
checked with her eye doctor and was told to go to the
emergency room if it happened again. In December it did.
The doctors contact Dr. Brooks at the University and because
of our family history a CT brain scan is followed with a MRI.
Damage to the brain, lesions, are found.

The end of May brings me to the University clinic with my
older sister. We have back to back appointments.

With the new information, the plan can now be more specific,
as the MRI's have now confirmed that there is something
going on in both my older sister and me. Because of this, we
are told we may have a familial disease. Dr. Brooks' fear
being it might be a "Buelah Baum Disease." But he now
knows what questions to ask and where to look for the
answers. He is attending a genetics group meeting in France.

The surprise on Mama's autopsy was the confirmation of
small strokes (vascular) along with Alzheimer's Disease. It is
our goal to stop our progression before the full Alzheimer's
manifests. The blood thinner, Plavix, is added for the
prevention of strokes. It is also not unreasonable to
associate the small strokes to the brain with small strokes
to the heart, thus my heart symptoms.

We have now moved from "limbo" into the genetics circle.
I re-contact the Alzheimer's Disease Research Center,
Seattle, Washington. She appreciates the update.

Thoughts...

Without my older sister developing her symptoms, I would still be in a "questionable" disease. How can I feel grateful and sad at the same time? Because it was found so early for her, little damage is done. Perhaps that can be my gift back to her. And with the two of us together, others in our family have a better chance to be healthier.... and that is our gift to them.

Spring 2001

Mama is moving away from me, no longer hanging tight by. There must be new events happening - she no longer sees the need to guide so close.

June 2001

I have had the greatest experience since the beginning of this long road. I have been proven right. They can believe me...

I am meeting with the neuropsychologist from the Memory Center, he happens to be the same doctor I saw for a brief visit in 1996. He has continued his education in dementias with classes every year. While at the Memory Center their focus is memory, he likes to evaluate all functions, such as: Is the brain retrieving the information that is stored effectively? He starts right out telling me that because of the Parkinsonian symptoms it would be evident that the basil gangula is affected. This is also where the brain retrieves and organizes the information - the "computer" of the brain.

Problems in the basil gangula would produce slow retrieval, slow response to problems, slow movements, slow conversations, and slow analyzing. Using a model, he shows me the parts of the brain. The basil gangula has no large blood vessels, only small capillaries. So any small vessel vascular disease is likely to affect it. By the results of his extensive testing he states that the locations of the other strokes are affecting organization and planning.

I am impressed that he handles all the testing himself (not using a technician), very thorough, very gentle, and very encouraging. He notes that I am less anxious now that we have a "named disease" to work with (a lot of people are) compared to the last meeting we had in 1996. I am even more impressed that he remembers me. I relate how quickly he was able to explain what was wrong with me when all the neuropsychologists at the University said it was "all in my head due to depression." It upsets him to think that I had to go fifteen years without the right answer - when it was obvious with neuropsychological testing.

His report later states that my brain functions at less than 10% when attempting multi-tasked problems. (What task is not multi-tasked?) And he continues to add "her self-report of neurological and emotional symptoms shows no evidence of defensiveness, over-reporting, or emotional contribution to her neuropsychological complaints." I could not have read anything more beautiful!

"They" can now believe me.

August 25, 2001

I see it in her face. My sister, the fourth victim of this awful disease, Mother, Aunt, Self, Sister.

I understand now how I was so far out of control. I thought I was handling it so well. She is in the beginning. I want to help - to stop it - I haven't enough control yet... I haven't enough of the answers. I sit and watch and remember. I sit and feel what she is feeling. I'm beyond and back from that point. But I remember the months and years it has taken. I don't want her to have to take this trip too.

She listens to a simple story of how our brother was caught in a rip tide while swimming on vacation. Her face distorts, her emotions rise. She cannot think of anyone else in danger. Danger, uncertainty. Why now do those things (feelings) exaggerate beyond proportion?

What was once such a simple life. Planned from day to day, event to event. No longer firm on the ground beneath.
We are not even beyond the beginning, we have not entered the abyss, and yet it tears apart and disrupts.
Every event that was so easy... ... ... Maybe that's it!...

It doesn't take away the "all," it takes the "easy," the small.
One step at a time! Until there is no "all" left.
And that is how we fight it! Find the "easy" first.
Nutrition - oh that's too easy, can't be that! Can it?!!
Hormones - blood - rest - bliss - find all the easy parts;
put them together!
Find its "all" before it has ours!

Summer 2001

Information on *The Nuns' Stories* has made it into the news. It is an epidemiology study of Alzheimer's Disease conducted on 678 Catholic nuns started in 1986 by David Snowdon.

By researching their lives from the time they entered the convent to their death, a clearer picture of Alzheimer's Disease was obtained.

The findings give us hope... plaque and tangles were found in the autopsy of a brain, although no other signs of Alzheimer's were present during her life. What was the protection?

To date, the following is offered:

> Prevent head injury of any kind by use of seatbelts, and helmets.
>
> Prevent strokes by not smoking, exercising and regulating blood pressure.
>
> Nutrition with folic acid and antioxidants such as Vitamins C and E.
>
> Continue learning to build up nerve cells thus keeping ahead of any loss.
>
> Mind games will exercise your mental muscle.
>
> Keeping spirits high.
>
> Know your genetic susceptibility.

Look for *Aging With Grace* by David Snowdon (Bantam 2001) for the full story.

Thoughts...

Perhaps meditation/prayer should be added to the list.

November 2001 Family Letter

After six years from my original request we have been asked to send our initial family medical history to the top genetic research center in the U.S. Attached you will find this information. Because our family falls under a most unique form of Alzheimer's, we have not previously fit any of the studies. A new study on chromosome 4 shows promise, as it is a Parkinson/Alzheimer combination. Also on chromosome 4 is a blood anti-coagulant factor. This may correspond to the family history of strokes/heart and thyroid, along with the mini-strokes that Mary Kay and I have been experiencing.

The researchers are requesting records from any kind of neurological problem. Also I was told that the dementia may skip a generation. See the chart for what we have found so far.

Dr. Brooks has stressed again that, for our family, a routine head MRI, an EEG, and blood test for Protime (the time it takes for blood to coagulate - ours seems too fast, thus leading to strokes) is essential. If a family has a history of cancer, cancer screening is advised. We have a hereditary factor for mini-strokes (which are silent), and seizures. These are controllable and caught early, we are hoping to prevent the end – full strokes, heart disease or full Alzheimer's Disease. Early symptoms can be any of the following: dizziness, vertigo (where the room spins around you), random pain that may move about, weakness, fatigue, tremors, change in vision such as aura or blurred or change in field of view or brightness, slow recall of information, change in speed of learning, memory, fainting, numbness, harder to focus on more than one activity at a time, dreams of danger, anxiety, depression.

Basically, take information on what a full stroke would entail and minimize it – as mini-strokes are very subtle and silent. Because the strokes are mini the symptoms may not last long sometimes only minutes, and any damage may disappear as your body heals/recovers, but if they are not stopped it will compound and you will get as bad as I did. Because the damage is done in the small vessels it may also appear in any of the organs of the body.

Early detection = early control.
Having had a base line MRI and EEG will save months of waiting to get onto medication because the changes will show up when these tests are repeated.

The focus has changed over the last year to include early detection, because of the great advances in stabilizing. The cure will be in genetics, and that's where we are now headed.

Love

Chris

Family letter from our older sister:

December 23, 2001

I've been meaning to write this letter for several months. I have small vessel vascular disease. So does Chris. So did Mama before it developed into Alzheimer's Disease and possibly vascular dementia.

The **good news** is that now we know a lot more about what we're working with. And the medications Dr. Brooks has given me have stopped mine from getting worse. And Chris' medications are actually reversing her small vessel disease after it had gotten pretty bad.

What I want most to tell you today is **why I bother.** This is really a spiritual question, about the meaning of life. It is not exactly fun to report every possible symptom to Dr. Brooks, go through lots of tests, and take multiple medications. My motivation is not really to postpone my death as long as possible. I am motivated instead to avoid a repeat of Mama's several years of confusion, loss of sight, seizures, and inability to talk and move herself. I don't want that to happen to me if I can avoid it easily now. Even more so, I don't want my husband and children to see me or care for me for years like that. And most importantly, I feel called to help advance medical research so my children don't have to fear that they'll get dementia, muteness, seizures, etc. Mama is being an inspiration to me in this, as is Chris.

Small vessel vascular disease prevents some of our oxygen-rich blood supply from getting to small blood vessels in brain and/or heart. The tiny vessel dies for lack of oxygen, and we say a very tiny stroke has happened and a lesion may be seen on an MRI. Most of these tiny strokes or infarcts have no immediate noticeable effect, depending on where they are. But a build-up of these unnoticeable or very silent strokes in important locations can combine to cause plaques or tangles.

As might be expected, Chris and I show lesions in different areas and with different results. By chance, I have one in the frontal lobe of the brain, near my language center, which explains my increased difficulty finding words under pressure. I also show some tremor when thinking under pressure (an early "Parkinsonian symptom," but not Parkinson's disease). Most of my lesions are luckily in areas of no known brain function and are actually where surgeons enter to get to more sensitive parts of the brain.

We want to prevent ourselves from progressing into **Vascular Dementia.** As the Johns Hopkins report on Memory says

> *After Alzheimer's Disease, the most common cause of memory loss is Vascular Dementia - a disorder often resulting from a series of tiny stroke (infarcts) within the brain. Each infarct may be so small that it is inconsequential alone; however, the cumulative effect of many infarcts can destroy enough brain tissue to impair memory, language, and other intellectual abilities. Symptoms can also involve other brain functions: loss of bladder and*

bowel control (incontinence); a mask-like facial expression; and weakness or paralysis on one side of the body are thought to be non-cognitive hallmarks of Vascular Dementia.

This is what we want to prevent in any of us. I am doing very well as you can see:

1995 A couple of experiences of vertigo (room looks circling) with a head cold.

Nov 1999 I see lights across my vision for 20 minutes. I get my retina checked as fine. It's called a visual aura without headache and I should report if have another.

Dec 1999 I see lights again for 20 minutes and go to emergency room. A CT brain scan shows a small relatively new lesion in the front lobe of brain. The MRI the next day showed **two small lesions.**

Spring 2000 I am tested over the months for MS and an Alzheimer's Disease marker—both negative. I have dizziness from a spinal tap. An EEG shows a spike in front lobe. I am put on Tegretol. Another EEG a couple months later shows that the spike is exactly as it was, when healing might have been expected. I feel fatigue but I graduate from seminary and enjoy doing lots of physical work in the old house.

Fall 2000 An MRI shows I now have **nine lesions** in the brain. Mirapex (to reduce Parkinsonian tremor), more Vitamin E and baby aspirin are added to my regimen. I feel fatigue in evenings from the additional medications. I'm ordained!

Spring 2001 An MRI shows still the same nine lesions. We have stopped the disease!

Summer 2001 I have memory losses, leaving my keys and

losing objects. I am emotionally on edge. An anti-depressant is added because the heavy-duty medications may be causing physical depression, which in turn can cause memory loss. **Fall 2001** I am feeling much better and don't have much fatigue at all. I feel the anti-depressant working well with my medications. I ask to stop the Tegretol, but a recent EEG shows the same spike and I must stay on it to avoid seizures. **Dec 2001 I feel I have fine tuned my medications and my disease is arrested!**

Well, there are some preventative measures we should all take. I believe all sons and daughters of Buelah should routinely **eat high in protein,** take **Vitamins E & C, Baby aspirin,** and **Ginkgo Biloba.** Plus we should take at least one good **multi-vitamin with folic acid**. Please also ask for an EEG and a MRI if you have any neurological changes, like any bouts with vision change, headaches unusual for you, vertigo, fatigue, weakness, depression, tremors, dizziness, involuntary movements or sounds, seizure, lack of circulation to extremities, or memory loss.

We know that the form of dementia that Mama had may pass genetically to **half** of us children. It may appear in very different ways, including effecting the heart. And it may be complicated by any Parkinson's or other neurological illness on Papa's side (Uncle George—ALS). We may have strokes without high blood pressure or high cholesterol. But with prevention and investigation, all of us and all our children may lead healthy lives.

Love,

Mary Kay

dreams...

A girl was working on a wall size art project.

It looked like a series of dashes and dots.

When I looked closer I could see it was words and

spaces – she was copying the phone book onto the wall.

Why? An exercise in patience and control.

I go to this house often in my dreams:

It is an old house with dark paneling and lots of floors,

with odd steps and different levels.

It is hard to find my way around. I am seeking but never

finding before I wake up.

And then one time:

I am in the house, having walked around again.

It is a bit more familiar. I know I have been here before.

I open a door to my left, about shoulder high, there he sits.

He is old in body, but not in mind. He is my guide.

I know him and I feel content.

I never have that dream again.

Fall/Winter 2001

My night time dream guide has changed.

"He," an older male figure who often meets me

in my dreams, has been replaced with a "mother figure."

I have reached the end of the struggle.

I am on my way back.

Guardians of Life

My Child
They are called Guardian Angels
Protectors of Young and Old

But Know them by Name
As they are the Ones Who Loved You

Have Faith in their Being
Made strong by Love of the Past

Let their presence Comfort You
And their strength Hold You Safe

Trust in their Guidance
As they give Fate its Direction

Teach your Children in Love
So they too will Feel

Their...
Guardians of Life

January 2002

I appear to be "going through menopause" a bit at a time. Passion Flower and Red Clover are two herbs I add into my regimen.

I take one capsule of Passion flower in the evening before bedtime for a quiet sleep. I also hope it will calm my mood swings a bit.

Red Clover is a natural source of phytoestrogen, an estrogen balancer. I start with one capsule in the morning and one capsule in the evening.

I look into them for menopause, but find both are also helping with the healing, as they are also aids in degenerative diseases.

Passion Flower (Passiflora incarnata) A.K.A.: Passion Vine, Maypops, Purple Passion Flower.

Passion flower gets it name from the finely cut corona found in the center of the flower blossom. It resembles the Crown of Thorns given to Jesus.

For menopause, Passion flower helps with nervous insomnia, hysteria, crying and restlessness.

The anti-inflammatory properties aid in sleeplessness caused by brain inflammation.

Passion flower contains harmine and harmaline alkaloids, two effective anti-Parkinson's disease compounds.

Passion flower is helpful for the sciatica nerve.

Its calming effect helps

twitching

epilepsy

convulsions

muscle spasms

hyperactive children

back tension

pain

Aids in eye infection, eye strain and eye tension.

Passion flower supports nerves, eyes, circulation, intestines, female organs, muscles, skin and head.

Red Clover (Trifolium pratense) A.K.A.: Purple Clover, Wild Clover, Trefoil, Cow Grass.

Red Clover is highly nourishing. Thus helping with nutrition in healing especially chronic, degenerative disease.

It has been used as a cancer curative. By preventing new blood vessels from forming around the cancer tumors, the tumors starve with no blood supply.

Red Clover blossoms contain the trace element Molybdenum. Molybdenum can be found in the liver, kidneys, bone and skin helping to discharge nitrogenous waste. (A blood purifier.) Molybdenum helps with lactation in nursing mothers. When added with iron supplements, it increases hemoglobin formation, an aid for anemia.

Red Clover aids menopause by its calming properties. It also relieves menopausal sore joints, anxiety and energy loss. It helps with hot flashes by replacing depleted vitamin B's and C, magnesium and potassium. The phytoestrogen properties promote estrogen. Also a hormone balancer.

Aids in the prevention of stroke.

Has bone mending properties.

Restores vitality.

Red Clover aids the skin , helping with:

>   acne
>
>   boils
>
>   burns
>
>   psoriasis
>
>   skin cancer
>
>   skin disease
>
>   sores
>
>   eczema
>
>   leprosy
>
>   wounds

Red Clover's antibiotic properties help with infections.

Improves the circulatory system, the digestive system and the respiratory system.

Aids in :

>   bronchitis
>
>   coughs
>
>   wheezing
>
>   whopping cough

Red Clover supports the nerves, blood, liver, lymph, heart, feet, respiratory tract, skin, digestive tract, eyes, gall bladder, throat, kidneys, immune system, and urinary tract.

January - April 2002

One of the strongest allies a person can have is their pharmacist and the pharmacy staff. I came to realize this as the pharmaceutical companies combined and then decided to stop the manufacturing of some drugs.

"Like-drugs" are supposed to be the same, but there is no way two labs can make identical drugs, especially if one is a capsule and the other a tablet. And then there is the issue of price, unfortunately too many people are also familiar with these huge jumps. Several years back, my pharmacist researched and found a generic capsule form of Eldepryl at a price a little over the cost of the generic tablets. The capsule form works so much better than the tablet. With the pharmaceutical companies' merger the price of the capsules has gone from $70 to $274 for a one month supply. The medication that works the best is the non-generic capsule form at about $380 for a one month supply. I have no choice but to go back to the tablets at $50 a month.

I do not expect what happens next. I experience a total withdrawal - as the tablets prove not to be as strong as the capsules. My pharmacist is very supportive with additional research and helps me through the changes by having me try several brands before we find the right one.

I then increase the Gotu Kola to offset the difference in strength of the different brand (it also proves to be cheaper).

I am grateful that I have a pharmacist and staff who will also take the time to listen. I send them a "Thank-you" note so they know how much I appreciate their help.

June 2002
I read **BEYOND ASPIRIN   *Nature's Answer to Arthritis, Cancer & Alzheimer's Disease*** by Thomas M. Newmark & Paul Schulick. © 2000   Published by Hohm Press, PO Box 2501, Prescott, Arizona 86302 (800-381-2700)

Inflammation and controlling it has always been a strong factor in Alzheimer's Disease. Because of the side effects of aspirin therapy, it has been difficult to follow the doctor's advice with aspirin. My stomach feels like it is burning.

This book has offered an easier way for me to control the inflammation. But I never dreamed to what extent this inflammation had reached - far beyond the brain!

Pay special attention to Chapter 18 - Gotu Kola has shown to inhibit Abeta Brain Plaque. This is a "must read" book.

BEYOND ASPIRIN   Nature's Answer to Arthritis,
Cancer & Alzheimer's Disease

Thomas M. Newmark & Paul Schulick © 2000

Printed with permission from Hohm Press, Prescott, AZ

Linking Inflammation to: Arthritic type pain; Cancer of skin, breast, colon, prostate; "Stickiness of Blood" Thrombosis; Strokes – mini & cerebral; Digestion of fatty acids – cholesterol lipids; and Alzheimer's disease.

Introduction The enzyme cycloxygenase-2 is responsible for out of control inflammation. COX-2 inhibitors refer to compounds, both synthetic and natural, that have the ability to inhibit this enzyme. By January 2000, research showed these inhibitors were going to affect cancer, arthritis, and Alzheimer's Disease.

Chapter One Aspirin, ibuprofen and naproxen – all nonsteroidal anti-inflammatory drugs (NSAIDS) have been our only choice for chronic pain. Serious side effects have included ulcers, kidney damage, etc. In December 1998 FDA approved a "safe aspirin" called Celebrex and later Vioxx. These were hailed to have less side effects.

Chapter Two The disease condition of certain forms of arthritis are a result of too much inflammation. Osteoarthritis becomes exacerbated by inflammatory and associated processes. The problem is not with natural, balanced inflammation, but with excessive inflammation. The chemicals that stimulate this imbalanced destruction are by-products of a particular enzyme in the body called

cycloxygenase-2 (COX-2). Joint tissues in the body generally exist in a state of working equilibrium – between
tissue degradation and tissue recreation – until the by-
products of an over stimulated COX-2 enzyme can create
a condition of inflammation that destroys the balance.
Inflammation in itself is not a bad thing; the activity of the
COX-2 enzyme in creating inflammation is a normal,
natural part of the body responding to stress and challenge. However, when the COX-2 inflammatory process
is aggravated and over-stimulated we see destruction.
Inflammation of rheumatoid arthritis can be localized or
generalized, affecting the entire body causing symptoms
of loss of appetite, loss of energy and a powerful sense of
simply being "unwell."

Discovery: Sir J. Vane discovered that aspirin decreased
the production of inflammatory hormones, or chemicals,
called prostaglandins. Prostaglandins were known to be
created by the cycloxygenase enzyme. This was the key.
Once they knew that aspirin reduced inflammatory
prostaglandins, they could begin to solve the inflammation puzzle. But with chronic use of NSAIDS (aspirin, etc)
came severe bleeding & kidney damage. The NSAIDS
disrupted the formation of inflammatory prostaglandins,
but also inhibited the balancing and protective features of
the COX enzyme which was essential for proper kidney
function and for protecting the stomach.

Discovery: In 1991 the COX enzyme was actually two.

Both had the ability to metabolize, or burn, a particular fat in the body. COX-1 is responsible for maintaining house-keeping balance – homeostasis – in the kidneys and stomach. COX-2 an isoenzyme is responsible for the creation of inflammatory prostaglandins out of the fat called arachidonic acid. Researchers raced to locate a "silver bullet" that would disrupt the inflammatory Cox-2 without inhibiting the protective COX-1. Thus the development of Celebrex and Vioxx in 1998.

Chapter Three   Besides arthritis; cancers and Alzheimer's enter the picture. Arthritis does not appear to lead to cancer. The relationship is between the over-expression of COX-2 inflammation in organs and the existence of cancers in those body systems. Depending upon where the inflammation arises, as it relates to the strength and weaknesses of the particular person, different diseases can occur - cancers including prostate, breast, skin, bladder, lung, ovary.

Chapter Four   As the activity of COX-2 is inhibited some cancers appear to diminish. We are coming to understand that cancer cells use inflammation, born of COX-2, as a mechanism for survival and growth. Fueled by arachidonic acid, spread by the stickiness of blood platelets which are increased at the sight of inflammation, and stimulated by the production of thromboxane from arachidonic acid by COX-2, cancer is able to spread. People typically do not die from having cancer, they die from the spread of cancer. Once the cancer paradigm gets a strong foothold more dramatic traditional protocols must be use. Before that point, the preventative power of herbs should be advocated.

Chapter Five Celebrex and Vioxx are not the total answer. Will long term use cause problems?

Chapter Six The world of medical science has recognized the discovery of COX-2 and COX-1 as one of the most significant discoveries of the modern era. Herbs may work better with fewer side effects. The choice of COX-2 inhibiting herbs discussed is based upon the traditional use of herbs for inflammatory conditions. Included are ones that are readily available in a high quality form and are considered for both the observed pharmacological effect of the whole herb and its principal "phytochemical" parts.

Chapter Seven Green Tea   Contains salicylic acid, a naturally-occurring COX-2 inhibiting compound that was the basis for aspirin. Green tea has 51 anti-inflammatory compounds that prevent the onset and severity of arthritis and 15 anti-ulcer phytonutrients that inhibit or prevent ulcers. Also 400 anti-oxidant components for Alzheimer prevention (page 181). In addition, Mayo Clinic's recent study of green tea showed reduced cancer cells, inhibited cancer cell growth, nuclei fragmentation of cells, and cell death. Best to use in a broad-spectrum, full herb. In a combination with extracts of turmeric or ginger a three fold to eightfold increase in anti-tumor properties results.

Chapter Eight   Chinese Goldthread and Barberry   Are rich sources of berberine. Compounds in these plants inhibit COX-2. Has a history dating back to ancient Egypt in reducing inflammation associated with arthritic conditions. Various research from 1998-1999 show suppression of cancers of colon, bladder, human leukemia cells, skin tumors and malignant brain tumors. Has the ability to keep the blood unsticky, and not clotting, and is therefore protective of brain tissue when in conditions of cerebral ischemia (stroke) (see also page 191).

Chapter Nine   Holy Basil   "Significant COX-2 inhibitory effect." Containing ursolic acid and oleanolic acid as some of its phytonutrients. A cancer preventative, including leukemia. It is antimutagenic, radioprotective (from radiation) protects DNA mutation, anti-tumor in human skin and increases the detoxification enzyme glutathione S-transferase a detoxifying cancer-protective enzyme. Affording brain protection by being a stress and cortisol reducer (see also page 231).

Chapter Ten   Turmeric   Research in NY Presbyterian Hospital and Weill Medical College of Cornell University reported in 1999 that the phytochemical, curcumin, in turmeric inhibited the activity of COX-2. Anti-tumor, anti-inflammatory, and anti-oxidative. Stimulation of liver and relief of digestive inflammation. May be ingested or applied topically. Stops the cellular suicide of brain cells when amyloid plaque becomes inflamed (see also page 186).

Chapter Eleven   Baikal Skullcap A rich source of the flavonoid, baicalein. Skullcap restores physiological balance both by inhibiting COX-2 inflammation and promoting the healing of damaged tissue through its powerful wound-healing properties. An inhibitor of nitric oxide. A strong anti-oxidant in that it is used immediately after a heart attack. Contains high concentrations of melatonin, and is a cerebral free radical scavenger (page 182).

Chapter Twelve   Hu Zhang – Solomon's Seal Nature's richest known source of resveratrol (red grapes and wine are noted for this) anti-arthritic, anti-cancer and heart protective. Scientists at Memorial Sloan-Kettering Cancer Center reported in 1998 that resveratrol is a powerful suppressor of COX-2 cancer promotion. Recently, scientists at Un of Illinois Dept of Surgical Oncology found resveratrol also restores glutathione levels, supporting cancer detoxification in the liver as well as stimulates the production of powerful and natural free-radical scavengers.

Chapter Thirteen   Rosemary   See also Chapter 18 Used to improve concentration and memory and to relieve headache. The topical application of oils of rosemary relieve aching, rheumatic muscles. French studies in 1992 showed ursolic acid, a constituent of rosemary inhibited arachidonic acid metabolism in human platelet and leukemia cells. Rutgers University researchers, in 1994, showed rosemary extracts inhibited processes that are known to fuel the growth of tumors. Components of COX-2 inhibitors were unearthed in 1998. Rosemary has anti-tumor, anti-oxidant, anti-mutagenic properties, immune system enhancement. It is recommended that extracts of the whole rosemary leaf be used.

A Broad Spectrum: The inflammatory COX-2 enzyme is encoded within our DNA and manifests throughout the body. Its imbalances can ravage multiple organ systems and lead to disability, dementia and death with its infinite number of visible and invisible manifestations. Thus the need for a broad-spectrum weapon.

Chapter Fourteen   Ginger   Considered a universal medicine – have to date located over 477 constituents. Ginger has multiple constituents that inhibit COX-2 and inhibit the 5-lipoxygenase metabolism of arachidonic acid, and thus deprive prostate cancer cells of their fuel for growth. Anti-tumor, anti-heat, balances reduction of inflammatory prostaglandins which regulate production of compounds that dilate the arteries. Restores healthy platelet function by inhibiting thromboxanes, a pain-reducer, and anti-ulcer. Contains melatonin for activity and sleep (melatonin is also found in the brain) and has 180 times more protein-digesting enzymes than papaya. Helps in regeneration of tissue. Not only safely modulates COX-2, but also safely brings balance to the COX-1 enzyme activity in a manner that is vastly superior to the synthetic NSAIDS, like aspirin.

Chapter Fifteen   Oregano Has 4 known potent COX-2 inhibitors. With 31 anti-inflammatories, oregano has more recognized anti-inflammatories than any other herb. Inhibits platelet aggregation, prevents thrombotic – clotting – events like heart attack and stroke. And does not cause bleeding or ulcers. Can be applied directly to the skin and it goes directly into the bloodstream and body.

Chapter Sixteen   Feverfew Used for fevers and depression. One of nature's richest botanical sources of melatonin. Multiple COX-2 inhibitors. Is anti-thrombotic which works to inhibit blood platelet aggregation (thickening) to prevent heart attack and stroke. Anti-inflammatory. Migraine preventative. Powdered form will break down – use in resinous form.

Chapter Seventeen   Hops   Inhibits the body's re-absorption of bone – aids in bone density and arthritic joints, eases pain, anti-inflammatory, chemo preventative against breast and ovarian cancer and leukemia cells. Induces sleep. Demonstrates significant COX-2 inhibiting effects.

Chapter Eighteen   COX-2 Inhibition & Alzheimer's Disease Rosemary, rich in ursolic and carnosic acids, is a potent COX-2 inhibitor. There is now compelling evidence that COX-2 inhibitors reduce brain inflammation and thus reduce the ravages of Alzheimer's Disease.

The brains of patients with Alzheimer's Disease show, in specific regions, the accumulation of plaque comprised of beta-amyloid peptides. The medical challenge is presented by the complications that can result from the body's inappropriate response to plaque (tooth decay, gum disease, stroke and heart attacks.)

The presence of senile plaque does not in itself mean that a person has Alzheimer's disease. The plaque on its own does not cause dementia, but triggers inflammation in the brain that can be avoided or reduced by anti-inflammatory agents.

An herb called Gotu Kola, used for thousands of years to promote mental clarity and brain function, not only works as an anti-inflammatory and relieves mental fatigue, but it inhibits Abeta brain plaque.

The filamentous brain lesions that define Alzheimer's Disease consist of senile plaque and neurofibrillary tangles. Swiss researchers found the curly fibers and tangles were also present in the liver, pancreas, ovary, testes and thyroid. The results suggest there are irritants throughout the body and one manifestation of the irritation is in the brain.

The unchecked inflammation is the cause of neuronal death. COX-2 indicators increased in rats' brains after oxygen deprivation. Rats treated with a COX-2 inhibitor had a higher survival rate of brain neurons after the oxygen deprivation.

By reducing systemic inflammation on a long-term basis, evidence is overwhelming that we can reduce the incidence or severity of Alzheimer's Disease.

Chapter Nineteen   Free-Radical Damage and Alzheimer's Disease

It is necessary to address both the inflammation and the oxidative stress in an Alzheimer's brain. Something is being created in the inflammation COX-2 process that is killing neurons. There is overwhelming evidence that free radicals of oxygen, thrown off in the inflammatory process, are responsible for neuronal death and brain impairment. Scientists at the University of Kentucky discovered that Alzheimer's brain tissue had oxidized DNA, oxidative stress byproducts in neurofibrillary tangles and senile plaque, and lipid peroxidation byproducts in the brain and spinal fluid.

Although Vitamins C & E are antioxidants, the multiple antioxidative capabilities of ginger with up to 500 known constituents; of green tea with over 400 constituents; and the powerful skullcap will provide a multiple phyto-chemical direction. These will laud COX-2 protection against conditions such as arthritis and cancer.

Chapter Twenty   Other Phytochemical Strategies for Dealing with Brain Plaque & Related Inflammation

There can be many imbalances or disturbances at work in creating the mental deterioration, a "syndrome" of the disease. Besides controlling inflammation , consider these four additional connections between COX-2 inflammation and Alzheimer's disease.

1. Beta-amyloid Plaque Inhibition / Toxicity Strategy

Asiatic acid inhibits the formation of Abeta plaque and that chemical is naturally present in Gotu Kola. Turmeric and ginger have the ability to abolish cellular suicide of cell death.

2. Beta-amyloid Wound Healing Strategy

It is the wounds of inflamed plaque, joint tissue in arthritis, and tissue assaulted from cancer that need to heal. Gotu Kola stimulates collagen formation, and promotes wound healing processes. (Can be used topically)

3. The Curious Nitric Oxide Strategy

In 1998 scientists concluded that nitric oxide is a chemical "messenger molecule" that flits about the body at speeds almost too fast to measure. It is believed to play a role in a number of bodily functions, including the regulation of brain activity, and facilitates the maturing of thought into action. Scientists theorize that nitric oxide imbalances are unhealthy and likely to be at the root of many disease conditions, and it spikes at points of inflammation. Brahmi is linked to the release of nitric oxide.

4. Cerebral Thrombosis / Berberine Strategy

An inflammatory hormone thromboxane promotes blood platelet stickiness. Chinese researchers in 1995 concluded the constituent, berberine, from barberry and Chinese goldthread, has the ability to inhibit the formation of thromboxane. Thus a protective herb for stroke.

Chapter Twenty-one   Omega-3: A Complement to Herbal Inhibition of Inflammatory COX-2

Omega-3 fatty acids are the basis for cell membranes and creation of hormones. The building blocks of life. When we eat the essential and other fatty acids, we incorporate them into our cell membranes. If we eat the correct fatty acids, our cellular membranes are strong, flexible, and discriminating. Omega-3's are in two forms, DHA and EPA. Having too little DHA in the brain is associated with cognitive decline during aging and Alzheimer's Disease. The body will create EPA from DHA. Omega-3 allows improvements in cancer and rheumatoid arthritis. Flaxseed oil, salmon oil, and algae are sources of Omega3.

Chapter Twenty-two Topical application, Aromatherapy

The skin is the largest organ in the body. Any compound that can penetrate the skin passes directly into the bloodstream without being neutralized or diluted by the liver with ingesting. A lower dose can be more effective. Ginger, turmeric, green tea, holy basil, rosemary and skullcap have been proven topical inhibitors of COX-2, also cancer inhibitors.

Aromatherapy – the essential oils stimulate the sensitive nerve receptors in the nose and sinuses. The "message" of the herb goes directly into our consciousness.

Black Pepper – for muscle fatigue, arthritis, neuralgia, Fibromyalgia and pain relief.

Spike Lavender – paralyzed limbs, stiff joints and sprains

Lemongrass – anti-inflammatory, muscular pain, pain relief, antipyretic and a relaxant

Rosemary – anti-inflammatory, memory loss, alertness, anti-depressant, enhancing neuromuscular tone

Chapter Twenty-three

Use broad spectrum herbal extracts

Do not look for components – Use the full herb.

Use the herbs together – they magnify each other's effects.

Can be used on their own – start with one, add more in, or change combinations.

Cook with herbs, drink tea, take a bath with herbs, take as a supplement, use in lotions and oils.

Watch for chemical extraction – no hexane.

Supercritically extracted, use of pressurized CO_2, is good.

For health and balance – drink water, exercise, eat wholesome foods, laugh, sunlight, garden, seek knowledge, love, use support, silence – bliss.

June - August 2002   Very Important!
"The skin is the largest organ in the body. Any compound that can penetrate the skin passes directly into the blood-stream." *Beyond Aspirin* Chapter 22 (page 197 this book*).*

Putting shredded ginger, green tea, rosemary leaves, and Gotu Kola leaves into a tea ball, I make a tea in a 2 quart container and dump the tea into my full bath water and enjoy a relaxing soak. The anti-inflammation and healing properties enter directly through my skin and into my bloodstream.

I have been having trouble swallowing - it felt like a pocket of phlegm was always in the top of my throat and I slept with an elevated bed. During the first night after the bath I awake because I literally feel my throat opening up - I try to cough and my throat is clear. I sleep very well.

I do not expect this - and it is only the beginning!
After several more soaks, swallowing liquids is easier, the swelling in my legs lessons - I can see bones. My upper arms that were shapeless and ugly "fat" (I kept them hidden) are more normal with muscles showing.

And then my face - which was very full, lacked expression, with a stiff smile (I could hardly look in the mirror) is changing with cheekbones and only one chin! My whole body had been swelling up - including my intestines.

I can only speculate on the changes in my brain!

June 2002

An article in the newspaper catches my attention. The Wisconsin Alzheimer's Institute at the University of Wisconsin, Madison, Medical School is setting up a registry for research. I call the number and leave my name and address.

June 24, 2002

A letter arrives from the Institute. The program is named The Wisconsin Registry for Alzheimer's Prevention (WRAP). The purpose is to identify adult children of persons with Alzheimer's Disease who might be willing to participate in research that may help find ways to delay or prevent the onset of Alzheimer's Disease in the future.

To participate, a diagnosis of Alzheimer's Disease must be verified by a review of medical records. That will not be a problem for our family.

I make photo copies of the letter and see that each of our family members receives a copy. I then talk with each one to see which will be interested. I go ahead and submit a copy of Mama's records and autopsy for our family. And then we await a reply.

July 2002

Last night was the wake for one of our contemporaries. She had cancer for 7 years. Today I realize - as I fall apart - that I am envious of her. She... laying in the casket, no hair, body ravaged with disease, a part of what she had been...
but her struggle is over.
I am envious that her struggle is over.
I am so tired of fighting.
So tired of trying to find the next step.
So tired of hiding my limitations.
So tired of hurting my family.
So tired of being a burden...
Three swift years and my family's pain would dissolve.
They would remember only the good.
I head out in my car, not sure where to go. I stop driving because I can no longer contain the tears. I ask my mother for help... again.

I see a hawk fly overhead. I am reminded of the day our mother died. I drive to the bookstore. Walking into an aisle of books - there in front of me is a book with the name "Buelah" in the title. Next to it a book with "German" in the title. I laugh and say "OK, I will continue to believe and never doubt your strength." Our mother's name is Buelah Rose.

She sends me home with Dr. Christine Northrup's *The Wisdom of Menopause.* Reading it helps me to settle through some of the turmoil.

July - August 2002
We are given a chance to find the "**Why.**"
I receive a phone call from the University of Washington Alzheimer's Disease Research Center. There has been a review of the records we have submitted at the end of 2001.

Great news! We fit their profile and they are ready to take blood samples for the genetic studies. It is very easy to achieve through a local lab. Ellen takes down the information and sends off a consent form for me to sign and send back. She contacts a local lab and sends them the information they need.

The blood is drawn on August 13th. I explain to the technician drawing the blood, straight off, that I am usually a hard draw. She apologizes for the fact that they are requesting four vials. I reply that we will do whatever it takes to get the full amount. The future of our family is in those vials.

Surprisingly, the draw is very quick and easy, the vein is a very good size - the first time in years and years, maybe +15 years! My last blood draw at the University in May took two technicians and they ended up using the top of my hand.

The herb tea baths are working!
The reduction in inflammation has allowed the veins to expand to a normal size.
This is a double good day!!

August 4, 2002

National News, *The Post-Crescent*

Scientists find key heart-disease risk

  Inflammation more of a factor than cholesterol

Boston   In the past year or two, experts say, the evidence has become overwhelming that inflammation hidden deep in the body is a common trigger of heart attacks, even when clogging in the arteries is minimal.

A validation of the information in *Beyond Aspirin, Nature's Answer to Arthritis, Cancer & Alzheimer's Disease* by Thomas Newmark & Paul Schulick.

October 2002

We have just received word that Mama's sister, Mabel, has passed away. She, too, has been suffering with Alzheimer's disease. Her family is out of state, so we hold a family Memorial for those family members who cannot travel.

She is a younger sister so her family is younger than ours.

Perhaps we will have answers for them too.

December 2002
Our daughter has a question about amino acids. I look
in the books I have, but do not find an answer. So I set off
to the book store. I am unable to find the information I
want but do end up with a book, although I keep putting it
back and don't know why I am getting it.

Excitotoxins The Taste that Kills
by Dr. Blaylock, Neurosurgeon
Health Press, PO Box 37470, Albuquerque, NM 87176

It describes a link between MSG, NutraSweet©, L-cysteine
and brain damage and neurological diseases. I thought we
were buying only what we thought was good, but these
additives are in so much more! I know I am sensitive to
NutraSweet©, perhaps these additives were adding to my
inflammation - or worse.

May be one more environmental puzzle piece.
The date I found this book - December 12th, our mother's
birthday.
Another gift from her.

I strongly recommend the reading of this book in full.

EXCITOTOXINS The Taste that Kills

By Russell L. Blaylock, M.D. ©1997

With permission, Health Press Albuquerque, NM

Russell L. Blaylock, MD is a board-certified neurosurgeon. A clinical assistant professor at the University of Mississippi Medical Center. In March of 1989 his father succumbed to the ravages of Parkinson's disease. Thus he began on his journey to help others avoid this terrible experience, resulting in the writing of this book. For the past sixteen years he has had a private neurosurgical practice, treating many cases of neurodegenerative diseases.

Excitotoxin: a substance added to foods and beverages that literally stimulates neurons to death, causing brain damage of varying degrees. Can be found in such ingredients as **monosodium glutamate (MSG), aspartame (NutraSweet©), cysteine, l-cysteine, hydrolyzed protein, and aspartic acid**.

Could effect how your children's nervous systems are formed during development so that in later years they may have learning or emotional difficulties, or damage the part of the brain known to control hormones. Artificial sweetener in diet sodas may also cause brain tumors. Excitotoxins could aggravate or precipitate neurodegenerative brain diseases: Parkinson's, Huntington's, ALS, and Alzheimer's. Especially at risk if you have had a stroke, brain injury, brain tumor, seizures, hypertension, diabetes, meningitis or viral encephalitis.

Labeled: MSG can be labeled any of the following

MSG	Hydrolyzed vegetable protein
Plant protein	Natural flavorings
Spices	Plant protein extract
Sodium caseinate	Calcium caseinate
Yeast extract	Textured protein
Autolyzed yeast	Hydrolyzed oat flour

MSG found in: (MSG may be in and unlabeled)

Malt extract	Malt flavoring
Bouillon	Broth
Stock	Flavoring
Natural flavoring	Seasoning
Spices	Natural beef or chicken flavor

Additives: (MSG may be in and unlabeled)

Carrageenan	Soy protein concentrate
Enzymes	Whey protein concentrate
Soy protein isolate	

Hydrolyzed vegetable protein is manufactured by boiling vegetables in sulfuric acid, neutralizing the acid with caustic soda and drying the resulting brown sludge. Additional MSG may be added. Watch for it in barbecue sauces and fast foods, or a creamy version in canned and instant soups, salad dressings and sauces. Not only does this contain three powerful brain cell toxins – glutamate, aspartate, and cysteic acid, but also several carcinogens. FDA does not regulate hydrolyzed vegetable protein.

Chapter 1: How the Brain Works (A review of the brain and how each part works.) Too much or too little of certain critical nutrients can adversely effect the brain. It is very resilient, but can be sensitive during development, when the intricate circuits are being formed. Injuries during the formation period can result in devastating effects years later.

Chapter 2: Amino Acids (How food is broken down and utilized. What is an amino acid, types, and receptors.) Amino acids are the chemical building blocks used to create proteins. Humans possess about twenty different types of naturally occurring amino acids which are supplied from either plant or animal proteins. Glutamate, aspartate, and glycine are three amino acids the brain uses unaltered. They are classified as excitatory transmitters and are involved in activating a number of brain systems concerned with sensory perception, memory, orientation in time and space, cognition, and motor skills. The brain depends on a delicate balance of excitatory and inhibitory systems.

Chapter 3: Exciting Cells to Death (Too much Excitotoxins. Effect on the developing brain. How they work. Free radicals. Excitotoxins and brain cell energy. Bias in research.)

*Japanese used a seaweed-based flavor-enhancer for thousands of years.

*In 1909 Dr. Ikeda found glutamate to be the chemical

enhancer – monosodium glutamate and processed it.

*American soldiers spoke of the great tasting Japanese rations. In 1948 the Armed Forces with manufacturers (Pillsbury, Oscar Mayer, Libby, Stokley, Campbell Soups, Continental, General Foods, and Bordens) purchased MSG from the Ajinomoto Company.

*In 1957 studies showed damage occurs from excess MSG and aspartate.

*In 1968 found widespread destruction of neurons in the hypothalamus and circumventricular organs - most severe in immature or newborn animals. Hypothesized this area did not have a blood brain barrier system.

*Hypothalamus regulates growth, onset of puberty, endocrine glands, appetite, sleep and wake patterns, biological clock and consciousness itself. Many effects did not appear until years later. Is associated with an early onset of puberty.

*Public was unaware that large doses were in baby food.

*MSG was removed from baby foods in 1969 by congress. However, no warning was given to pregnant women and the danger of MSG to the fetus.

*A child's brain is four times more sensitive than an adult to excitotoxins.

*Glutamate and aspartate are neurotransmitters found normally in the brain and spinal cord. When their concentrations rise above a critical level, they can become deadly toxins to the neurons and nerve cells.

*High doses cause destruction within minutes. Lower doses seem to delay the destruction for several hours and then suddenly act.

*Vitamins E and C, K, D, A, and beta-carotene, magnesium, chromium, zinc and selenium help to offset the damage.

*The neurons are extremely sensitive to the toxic effects of glutamate and aspartate when cell energy is low. So hypoglycemia or low blood sugar plays a vital role in excitotoxins. (Diet soda on an empty stomach.)

*FDA? Both research and subcommittee reports have been compiled by The Glutamate Association, the manufacturers. (They want their food to taste best.) The studies were set up in such a way to prove MSG safe, although independent studies showed it was not.

Chapter 4 Effect of Excitotoxins on the Developing Brain   Glutamate is essential to brain development in the fetus.

It is suspected that brain development continues into adulthood, making newborns and toddlers at a very high risk when exposed to excitotoxic food additives. Because the brain continues to repair itself (plasticity), adult brains are also sensitive to an excessive amount of glutamate.

*Excitotoxins can cause excessive electrical activity of the brain and can cause seizures.

*By interfering with the timing of the stages of the development of the brain possible damage may be done which will show up as learning disorders, emotional illness or major psychological disease later in life (dyslexia, frequent outbursts of uncontrollable anger, autism, schizophrenia, seizures, cerebral palsy).

*Each exposure may kill some brain cells – and over many years a point is reached where the effects of the loss become obvious.

*One study seems to indicate that certain amino acids not only pass through the placenta, but also concentrate on the fetal side of the circulation. This means that the baby is exposed to a higher concentration of the amino acid than the mother is.

*We are not born with an intact and functional blood-brain barrier system. There is some evidence that it may not reach complete maturity until adolescence. During this period of growth and development the nervous system is particularly vulnerable to the damaging effects of a multitude of excitotoxic compounds (MSG, aspartate NutraSweet©, etc). During these formative years is when our children crave "junk food," the very type of processed foods that contain the highest concentration of excitotoxin taste enhancers.

*Some people lack the critical enzymes altogether needed for protection against excitotoxins in the diet. (From a study on ALS, Lou Gehrig's Disease.) One such enzyme (glutamate dehydrogenase) functions to convert glutamate into a harmless compound.

*This enzyme has been found to be defective in some neurodegenerative disorders. When these individuals eat diets containing MSG their blood levels of glutamate rise much higher than a normal person, and remain high for prolonged periods of time. This defect is present from birth, others may have less of the enzyme. They may be unaware of this biochemical defect.

*Immature brain cells exposed to excitotoxins can show a time dependent loss of the cellular antioxidant glutathione. It is the anti-oxidants that protect the cells once the sequence of destructive events is triggered by the excitotoxins.

*Vitamin E has been shown to significantly block the toxic effect of glutamate in brain cell cultures.

*Hypoglycemia (low blood sugar) and hypoxia (low oxygen) can greatly increase the damage done by excitotoxins. It takes energy to utilize the enzyme that converts glutamate into a harmless compound. Glutamate and aspartate will build up in an energy-deprived brain and kill the cells.

*Other neurological conditions are found to be related to excessive excitotoxin exposure, such as hypoglycemia, head injury, migraine headaches, seizures, and possibly the neurodegenerative diseases.

*The food industry was regularly adding MSG to baby foods from 1949 – 1969 in large enough concentrations that one jar contained enough to do damage to the brain.

*Watch for the compounding effect: a single frozen diet food dinner may contain MSG, hydrolyzed vegetable protein, and natural flavoring. Add in a diet drink with NutraSweet©, and low blood sugar (hypoglycemia), wow!
*Effects on Hormones: (endocrine system) (Damage to the arcuate nucleus of the hypothalamus.) Regulates the amount of hormone-releasing factors secreted by the hypothalamus and the pituitary which controls the release of hormones from the endocrine glands through-out the body – such as the thyroid gland, the adrenal glands, and the gonads.
*Problems: Obesity – that people cannot diet away (compounded with aspartate in NutraSweet©), reproductive problems in both men and women, early onset of puberty, lower thyroid hormone levels and higher cortisone levels than normal, could act as the trigger for diabetes in genetically susceptible people.

Chapter 5: Creeping Death: Neurodegenerative diseases.
What causes particular neurons to start dying after decades of normal function? What is causing neurons to slowly die? Why are only certain neurons susceptible to this death while neighboring neurons remain perfectly healthy?
*Most impressive line of investigation is the possibility of an environmental factor in genetically susceptible people.
*Along with low energy (famine), low magnesium which increase the toxicity of excitotoxins.

*Herbicides Cyperquat and Paraquat play a role.

*Parkinson's Disease - Glutamate, amphetamines and other excitotoxins may produce Parkinsonism by overexciting cortical glutamate cells that connect to the nigrostriatal neurons lying deep in the brain.

*L-DOPA is a mild excitotoxin so persons with Parkinson's disease should avoid all foods and drinks containing excitotoxin additives such as MSG, hydrolyzed vegetable protein, cysteine, and aspartate, etc.

*There are several conditions under which the blood-brain barrier system will fail: head injuries; viral and bacterial infections of the brain and spinal cord; hypertension; exposure to some metals such as lead and tin; an elevated core body temperature; and, major and minor strokes.

*Recent evidence that Parkinson's patients have a defect in their metabolism which leads to an increased metabolism so their resting energy expenditure is high, causing low blood sugar and low energy to the brain more often. Thus more vulnerable to excitotoxin damage.

*Patients with Parkinsonism seem to have an enzyme (Complex I-NADH = ubiquinone oxidoreductase) defect affecting only certain brain cells in the substantia nigra. This prevents these neurons from producing adequate amounts of energy.

*Within all cells energy is supplied by the mitochondria, which occurs via a series of reactions involving various enzymes and chemicals called the electron transport system. The first and most critical step in this energy producing process is called complex I. The neurons become severely depleted of energy and as a result become extremely sensitive to excitotoxins.

*We know that when glutamate over stimulates a neuron it can damage the mitochondrial genetic material, which would then pass on this altered gene to other cells.

*There are more diseases having a mitochondrial DNA defect inheritance rather than the usual chromosomal DNA defect inheritance.

*Parkinson's patients with continued exposure to MSG, aspartame, etc. may damage other neurons leading to symptoms of Alzheimer's type dementia and ALS.

*Parkinson's disease is affected with lower doses of excitotoxins spread over a longer period of exposure. ALS (Lou Gehrig's Disease) is seen with an exposure of more massive doses of excitotoxins in a shorter time period.

*ALS is a neurodegenerative disease that primarily affects the anterior horn cells of the spinal cord and the corticospinal tract. It can be present in many different forms. High serum glutamate levels are seen. Some have a defect in the enzyme glutamate dehydrogenase, also may have a deficiency of glutamate transporter proteins (removal of free glutamate), also may have a defect in the antioxidant enzyme – super oxide dismutase (SOD).

*L-leucine, magnesium, zinc, antioxidants such as vitamin E, supplements that increase cellular glutathione levels are preventatives. Avoid foods with excitotoxins.

*Huntington's Chorea: Damage to basal ganglion small and intermediate sized neurons, with almost complete sparing of the larger neurons. The degree of low brain metabolism varied directly with the stage of the disease. Glutamate imbalance related.

Chapter 6 Alzheimer's Disease: A Classic Case of Excitotoxin Damage

Experiments have shown: first, glutamate can induce the same Alzheimer specific types of proteins in normal cultures and second, once the neurons begin to degenerate, they will form abnormal proteins in the form of beta-amyloid. This amyloid protein can further enhance the toxicity of glutamate and aspartate in a dose dependent manner, so that the more plaques that are formed (i.e. the higher the concentration of beta-amyloid) the more sensitive the surviving neurons become to excitotoxins.

*This would mean that further exposure to excess excitotoxins, both from food additives and from those normally within the brain itself, could accelerate the process causing the disease to progress more rapidly. (Cascade) Recurrent bouts of severe hypoglycemia can cause accumulated brain damage much like mini-strokes.

*Other factors in dementia: silent mini-strokes, low thyroid hormone production (hypothyroidism), depression, low brain levels of B12, fevers.

*The neurofibrillary tangles are primarily located in neurons having glutamate receptors. Analysis of the protein content reveals that glutamate and aspartate are found to be the highest concentration of any of the amino acid components

*In 1985, two scientists, working with spinal cord cells in tissue culture, discovered that prolonged exposure of the neurons to glutamate or aspartate (excitotoxins) resulted in the formation of paired helical filaments almost identical to those seen in Alzheimer's Disease.

Energy: The key to brain protection. The brain normally contains relatively low concentrations of glutamate and aspartate, which are used as metabolic fuels and as neurotransmitters. (Glutamate is the most common neurotransmitter in the brain.) But the concentration of these excitatory amino acids within the brain must be carefully regulated so as to prevent toxic amounts from building up around the neurons. To prevent this from happening, the brain possesses an elaborate system to prevent glutamate accumulation. It uses an energy dependent pump system that literally pumps excess glutamate into surrounding glia cells where it is deactivated by enzymes. If this protective system fails because of lack of energy, accumulated glutamate will lead to cell death.

*Low blood sugar (hypoglycemia) will cause lack of brain energy. Other causes are cutting off of the brain's blood supply by stroke.

*So less brain injury from chronic exposure to excess glutamate or aspartate will occur when one's diet contains adequate protein & carbohydrates. (Famine, dieting)

*Merely going without food overnight can greatly increase the toxicity of MSG.

*Not all areas of the brain transport and consume glucose at the same rate. The hippocampus has a much narrower margin between its supply and its needs than does the cerebellum. So when glucose is low it is the hippocampus that is injured first and most severely.

*Patients with Alzheimer's Disease consistently demonstrate low metabolism in certain parts of the brain.

*For the brain to receive an adequate amount of glucose on a constant basis three conditions are necessary.

First, glucose must be absorbed from the intestines and enter the blood.

Second, the glucose in the blood must be transported across the blood-brain barrier into the brain.

Third, the brain cells must be able to convert the glucose into usable energy, primarily ATP.

In Alzheimer's all three systems are impaired.

*Magnesium appears to play a vital role. It is involved in over three hundred enzyme reactions.

*L-cysteine has been found to cause the same pattern of neuron destruction. (In BREAD)
*Zinc works against L-cysteine.

What to Do? List of observations made that could possibly be applied to treatment and/or prevention

Avoid excitotoxin food additives. Watch for MSG (monosodium glutamate), hydrolyzed vegetable protein, and aspartame (NutraSweet©).

Free radicals play a major role. Reduce free radicals with vitamins C, E, and beta-carotene. Minerals selenium, zinc and magnesium.

Anti-inflammatory nutrients such as Omega 3 – fatty acids from flax seed oil or fish oils.

Anti-inflammatory nutrients may also restore the blood-brain barrier.

The brain is starved for energy, eat plenty of complex carbohydrates and some sugars as a mixed meal. (Try not to eat sugar alone especially in drinks.) Proteins – eat well!

Regular exercise – not aerobics.

Cellular metabolism appears to lie in utilizing L-carnitine, Co-Q10 and Vitamin C.

Magnesium and zinc are beneficial.

Caffeine is a mild brain stimulant, which increases metabolism and the need for more energy, which is impaired. Try to limit caffeine.

Chapter 7 Other Neurological Disorders
Related to Excitotoxins

Seizures: Complaints and evidence of seizures especially
after use of NutraSweet©

Magnesium and zinc reduce the chance of seizures.

Headaches: Number one complaint by consumers using
products containing NutraSweet©. Migraines are
seen with NutraSweet© and MSG use.

500 mg of magnesium lactate or gluconate daily
for one week and then a maintenance dose of
250mg a day thereafter works for migraine suffers.
Women who have migraines triggered by their
menstrual period – add in Omega 3 fatty acids, it
blocks the inflammation. Hypoglycemia will add
to migraines and tension headaches.

Brain Injury: Glutamate levels are elevated for days
following a brain injury.

The blood–brain barrier may be disrupted.

Watch: there is glutamate and aspartate in many of
the tube feeding formulas. (Bad) Some evidence
that treatment of spinal cord and brain injured animals with antagonist (excitotoxin blocking drugs)
of glutamate can reduce the severity of the injury.

Strokes: Ischemia-Anoxia: Pathological findings seen
with strokes closely resemble the selective neuron
damage observed with excitotoxins.

The neurons in the zone of infarction began to

increase their rate of firing before they died. Observed increased glucose metabolism in these dying and hyperexcited neurons. Observed significant elevation of excitatory amino acids, aspartate and glutamate in infarct region. Found that excitotoxin-blocking drugs greatly reduced the degree of neuron death. Glutamate-blocking drug MK-801. High doses of magnesium could protect neurons from prolonged periods of a lack of oxygen. Alcohol and phosphates significantly lower body magnesium levels. (Carbonated colas are high in phosphates.) Supply of brain energy will be low – sensitivity to MSG, aspartate, etc., will be high.

Hypoglycemia: The supply of energy to the brain and spinal cord cells plays a vital role in protecting cells from the damaging effects of excitotoxins. When hypoglycemia is severe, the brain's supply of ATP is rapidly depleted. This knocks out the mechanism the brain uses to protect itself from abnormal accumulations of glutamate and aspartate. Brain damage can be reduced by using drugs known to block the harmful effects of glutamate. Avoid simple sugars.

Brain tumors and AIDS: Levels of a powerful excitotoxin called quinolinic acid were twice to twenty times higher than normal in the cerebrospinal fluid of patients having AIDS.

Cell-mediated immunity is important in fighting viruses, bacteria and cancer. It was suggested that this defect in immunity was caused by damage to the hypothalamus induced by neonatal exposure to MSG. The hypothalamus plays a vital role in immunity. First experiments done to test safety of aspartame in **1981** disclosed a high incidence of brain tumors in the animals fed NutraSweet©.

A by-product of aspartame metabolism is diketopiperazine (DKP). When nitrosated by the gut it produces a compound closely resembling a powerful brain tumor causing chemical, N-nitrosourea. From 1973 to 1990 brain tumors in people over the age of sixty-five have increased 67% - with brain tumors in all age groups jumping 10%. The greatest increase in brain tumors has occurred during the years **1985, 1986, 1987.**

Use of aspartame has grown: 1985, 800 million pounds in U.S. Over 100 million people drink aspartame-sweetened drinks, including children. It has been suggested that the encephalopathy and dementia seen in the terminal stages of AIDS may be due to glutamate accumulation in the brain and not as a result of the virus itself.

Conclusion: Summary

*Excitotoxins can have a devastating effect on the nervous system in all stages of development – embryo to adult.

*Exposure during the developing brain of the infant and child, is linked to the later development of adult neurodegenerative disease.

*When MSG was first added to food, glutamate receptors had not been discovered. No one knew that excess glutamate could cause brain cell death.

*It was only after tons of these "taste enhancers" were being added to our foods and beverages that the discovery of serious side effects was made.

*This discovery remained buried in the medical research literature for over a decade before someone recognized this danger.

*Abundant research had demonstrated that these excito-toxins damaged the cells of the retina of the eye, and in the hypothalamus and other vital areas of the brain.

*The toxic effect of excitotoxins occur at a time when no outward symptoms develop, the child does not become sick or throw up or have any behavior to alarm parents that something is wrong.

*As the child develops, the damage may present itself as an endocrine disorder or even possibly a learning disorder (autism, attention deficit disorder, dyslexia) or an emotion control disorder (violent episodes, schizophrenia, paranoia).

*Through the efforts of Dr. John Olney, the food industry was forced to halt the use of excitotoxins in baby foods.

*No one warned pregnant mothers that the MSG laced food they were eating could endanger the fetus.

*MSG was added to virtually every processed food, and sold as an additive (Accent, etc.) for in home use, 1960's.

*In 1969, James Schlatter, a bench biochemist working with a compound called aspartame as a possible cure for stomach ulcers, happened to lick his thumb while turning a page in his notebook. Struck by the intense sweetness of the chemical, created NutraSweet©.

*In 1988 NutraSweet© reaped $736 million in sales.

*Despite concerns over the safety of this new sweetener, including brain tumor induction in experimental animals, seizures, precipitation of headaches, and an adverse effect on the developing brain, the FDA approved its use.

*FDA had recently outlawed cyclamate.

*FDA changed labeling laws so that the words "monosodium glutamate" is not required on food labels unless it contains 100% pure MSG.

*MSG need not even be mentioned by any name if one product containing pure MSG is only used as an ingredient in another food. If broth is used to make a soup, and the broth contains pure MSG, MSG does not have to be listed as an ingredient. But if the broth is sold alone, it must appear on the label.

*Substances labeled as "spices," "natural flavoring," and "flavoring," may contain anywhere from 30% to 60% MSG. The consumer is denied this information.

Chapter 8 Update

New information on the lethal effects of excitotoxins, and a growing list of ways to reduce the damage.

*"Excessive excitotoxin accumulation within the injured brain" constitutes the leading theory of a **final common pathway** for a multitude of disorders affecting the central nervous system, from strokes and trauma to neurodegenerative diseases and seizures.

*Aspartame increases the brain levels of phenylalanine and methanol. Methanol is converted within the brain tissues into formic acid and formaldehyde, both powerful neurotoxins. With aspartame, we have two neurotoxins plus an excitotoxin.

Part I

*Pharmaceutical Agents: (A full listing in the book.)

> Certain pharmaceutical agents are used to block glutamate toxicity – when the source is *within the brain.* Followed by an approach for – *excitotoxins entering the brain* from the blood stream: Arachidonic acid leads to eicosanoids, both good and bad. (Bad eicosanoids suppress immune function, impair BLOOD FLOW, and promote INFLAMMATION.)

*Nutritional Protection:

Besides reducing the concentration of excitotoxins themselves, there are three major areas in which nutritional supplements may help in preventing damage.

1. Reducing "Bad" Eicosanoids

> Diet: Connection between hypoglycemia, insulin, and "bad" eicosanoid production. Eat complex carbohydrates, lean protein, low saturated fats.

> Omega 3-fatty acids reduces the generation of arachidonic acid, reduces blood coagulation, improves cell membrane fluidity,
> blocks the production of "bad" type eicosanoids, improves nerve conduction within the optic nerve. Complement with Vitamin E.

2. Reducing Free Radicals: Effects of brain aging -

Free radicals can damage cell membranes, intracellular components, and mitochondria DNA. (Mitochondrial DNA affects only the involved mitochondria not the genetics of the cell itself – this defect is passed onto the new mitochondria when it reproduces. Takes many years to see the damage.)

> N-Acetyl L-Cysteine (NAC) (not L-cysteine the excitotoxin).

> Multiple antioxidants vs single – Use in combination to cover all types of free radicals. Vitamin E (dl and d), C, CoQ10.

3. Improving Energy Production: Once excess free radical
generation is corrected, we are still left with damaged
mitochondria that are unable to produce a sufficient
amount of energy for normal functioning and survival.

Coenzyme Q10 plus niacinamide – also riboflavin
and thiamine. Significant in preventing
damage.

Acetyl L-carnitine: antioxidant, increases
mitochondrial energy production, stabilizes cell
membranes, increases cholinergic transmission
in the brain (involved in memory), and chelates
iron. Shown to reduce and reverse brain aging.

L-Carnitine: Reduces the deteriorating histological
changes as well as slows down behavioral
deterioration. Improves long-term memory,
discriminatory learning, spatial learning and
seems to extend longevity. Improves cellular
energy production.

Taurine: Plays a major role in stabilizing nervous
system excitability. Manufacturers now adding
to infant feedings in hospitals.

*Further Improving Brain Function Nutritionally:

Lecithin: Improves memory by increasing the
availability of choline.

Also used to repair injuries to the insulation of
nerves (myelin sheath) in cases of MS, stroke
and head injury.

Phosphatidylserine: Improves memory function, a natural glutamate blocker, improves cell membrane stability and fluidity. Avoid products made from animal brains.

Hydergine (Dihyro-ergot compound): Helps economize the brain's ATP levels, thereby preventing a sudden drain on brain energy reserves during times of stress, offers membrane stability, improves alertness. Physician dosed.

DMEA (Deanol or dimethylaminoethanol) : Increases choline which increases acetylcholine. Reduced hyperactivity, increases attention span, reduced irritability (an alternative to Ritalin).

*Stabilizing the Blood-Brain Barrier:

Like the brain, the eyes have their own blood barrier system. Flavonoids or bioflavonoids can protect the eyes from damage by disease and aging. Some may also work for the brain.

Rutin – flavone

Querectin - flavone: found to be a potent and prolonged inhibitor of proinflammatory arachidonic acid metabolism.

Hesperidin – flavone: found to inhibit the enzyme (phospholipase A2) responsible for the release of arachidonic acid.

Alpha-lipoic acid: Reduced form DHLA (dihydrolipoic acid)

Is it a miracle nutrient?

Meets criteria for "universal antioxidant."

Regenerates other antioxidants as vitamin C and E.

Increases the levels of coenzyme Q10 (ubiquinol) during times of oxygen stress.

Increases intracellular antioxidant glutathione.

Is available to all tissues after dietary supplementation.

A free radical scavenger.

Ability to chelate free iron and copper. Complete protection against mercury and arsenic.

Diabetic polyneuropathy (disorder of arms & legs) was significantly improved.

Prevention of cataract.

Protection from mortality - stoke or cardiac arrest.

Improved performance on memory tests.

Alpha-lipoic acid (not DHLA) gives profound protection against radiation injury (Chernobyl disaster).

May prevent/reverse neurodegenerative diseases.

Works best if it is taken on a daily basis to build up preventative protection.

Part II – What Did the FASEB Report Really Say?

        Hidden truths.

Notes: All newer anti-seizure medications are glutamate blocking drugs.

        Infant feeding formulas contain very high levels of free glutamate especially those made from casein hydrolysates.

        MSG or aspartame is added to child related food products and medications - vitamins, cold preparations, vaccines, food.

        Virtually all of the neurodegenerative diseases are now considered to be intimately related to the excitotoxic process.

        Developmental brain disorders, seizures, headaches, strokes, brain injury, and subarachnoid hemorrhage are all intimately related to excitotoxins.

Reference to *Brain Repair* ...
This is not the first time we read about Excitotoxins. In *Brain Repair,* Chapter 4, (page 57 of this book) we see *blood-brain barrier, excitotoxicity, excess glutamate and aspartate.*

Thoughts...
The feelings of a backward slide has lessoned dramatically since eliminating as much of MSG and aspartame as I can. Like all foods and food sensitivity, it may not affect everyone. I had gone to the doctor for an uncontrollable itching when aspartame was first used in diet soda. He gave me some strong medicine, but didn't know why I was itching. I then found a small 2" column in a magazine, that stated some people are allergic to the new diet soda. The most common complaint was uncontrollable itching. So I know I am allergic to aspartame. Although I did not realize how "toxic" it would be for me and my family.

And if there has been damage to the blood-brain barrier, the likelihood of it occurring is much greater. One more cause for inflammation... One more puzzle piece.
This is one area where we can exercise prevention and be full of care for the next generation.

If the FDA requires "hidden" peanut warnings on all foods, for those who are allergic to peanuts, perhaps there can be a reconsideration on the lack of MSG labeling for us.

In the beginning, I had to keep my research broad, as we

were unsure of what disease we were looking at. And so I have read materials related to numerous diseases. There are two key elements found in Alzheimer's Disease, that are also in MS, ALS, Fibromyalgia, Arthritis, Cancer, Strokes, Huntington's, Parkinson's, Heart and other diseases.

First is INFLAMMATION out of control. The area of the inflammation will vary, but it is still inflammation.

Second is the damage from the EXCITOTOXINS. Again depending on the weakness of the body, the area of destruction by the excitotoxins will vary, causing different symptoms, but the destruction of cells is the same.

Perhaps with this knowledge, others will have clues to stopping the cascading effect of their disease.

How important has finding the books *Beyond Aspirin* and *Excitotoxins* been? They have changed my life!
The damage done throughout the past 15+ years has left my body ravaged. The pain, the weakness, loss of memory, the feeling of imbalance, foggy brain... will not be healed with the medications alone.

Over the months, using the information found in these books has been as important as the blood thinners and other medications. Until "they" find all the answers, it will take a combination of factors to stay ahead. The anti-inflammation and anti-oxidant herbs playing a major role.

My family has joined in, because of the hereditary factor and the unknown damage of the excitotoxins. Each are careful to omit all forms of MSG, and aspartate/aspartame. Perhaps by doing so, the next generation will not have to deal with this disease.

December 2002

If I were to summarize the year 2002 in one word it would be menopause. I'm at my family doctor's and ask about the "hot flashes" that seem to most occur when I am stressed. She states that is because they are serotonin based. I hadn't put that together before. We know that the level of serotonin is a factor in my disease.

I had often wondered why the medication I was on seemed to make my body "feel" as if it was getting younger - kind of like the fountain of youth. I was always kidding my family about it. Was this why I had "hot flashes" not related to menopause years ago, early in the disease process? Are the "hot flashes" that I am experiencing now menopausal or disease related? By cutting back on the medication, I seem to be proceeding on with menopause.

Our mother progressed at her worst when she went through menopause. (Perhaps because of the lack of serotonin and other hormones.) Although it was early in her descent, I think it was the scariest time. So menopause elicits a strong fear in me. Will I be able to hold my own?

Artisan of Life

Ribbons and bows, Glue and thread
Bits of treasures Past

Twisted wires, Skillfully formed,
Frames of Strength

Nature's Palette, Blended hues
Elegant loops and curves

Tenderly tucked, Knotted with Care
Images Unfold

Ever changing Ideas, Simply gathered
Secretly Patterned

Patiently held, Gently shaped
Knowing Hands Transform

Segments of Life, Held in Time
Molded in Love...
         Treasures of the Heart

January 2003

"I am a Survivor"

It all seems so simple now.

I was rereading my writings and journals and found that I have moved beyond so many of those feelings! Even a couple of months ago I would say the feelings still applied. Now I see them as "past" and I am sure that what I have done is important enough to share with others.

My credentials are that I am a survivor. I have been to age 90 and back. I have felt it all! With the knowledge and all the help our mother has given us, comes the responsibility to pass it on.

"She has always guided me. Her spirit is with me. She was a nurse and would never allow her children to go through what she did before she died. I believe this with my whole being."

"Just before the cure appears, almost every patient experiences a dramatic shift in awareness. He knows that he will be healed, and he feels that the force responsible is inside himself but not limited to him - it extends beyond his personal boundaries, throughout all of nature. The word that comes to mind when a scientist thinks of such sudden changes is *quantum.* The word denotes a discrete jump from one level of functioning to a higher level - the quantum leap."   *Quantum Healing, Exploring the Frontiers of Mind/Body Medicine* by Deepak Chopra, M.D. (Chapter II)

What does survivor mean to me? Physically, I have been able to slow or stop the progression enough to begin to heal. I am at a better place than our mother was during the same course of the disease. Spiritually, I am learning to live and love again, to feel a part of the universal energy. Scientifically, the answers will come only with my autopsy.

I relate my feelings to my brother.
"Given the opportunity to change things, would I travel this road again?" he asks.
I cannot see myself as whole without knowing what I do now. So, except for the hurt it has brought my family,
I would.
I have learned so much.
I have traveled roads I did not know existed.
Perhaps others will benefit....

January 24, 2003
I believe we have been through life before. Each time evolving to a higher level of goodness. Today I handed my daughter the first chapter of this book. She in turn handed me a print of the first ultra sound of their to be second child. The baby lay face up, tummy showing, legs and arms fully visible - all at 10 weeks.

Last night in starting on this book I realized I said I was a survivor the same month she felt she was pregnant.
Wouldn't it be nice if our mother's job is now over and she took that next chance for a new life?

February 2003

The journey back is hard - painful. At times I'm not sure
about it. You'd think it would not be a problem. Not so
much physical pain as mental pain. As you come back you
feel more. The ups become higher, the downs become
lower. You leave that "safe" mono feeling of numbness to
the world that took years to reach.

The steps forward are firmer. But there are always the
steps backward. And when that happens it hurts so bad.
The loss, although it may not look like much to someone
else, feels so great - so astronomical. I know this spot.
I know its limitations. I've been here before.
I feel its anguish. I feel its heartbreak.
I do not want to relive it again.
It is already a part of me, of my memory, of my being.
I thought I had gone beyond it.
I thought I was in a better place. Don't leave me here.
I have already tasted the better. I've already seen
over the hill.
Why do I have to climb it again?
It took so much energy, so much fortitude, so much
emotional strength to make each step.
And that backward slide?
It only took a moment.
Where do I find the ability to do it again?

March 13, 2003

USA Today

Painkillers May Dissolve Alzheimer's Plaque

Test-tube study lends hope, must face human trials.

The test-tube study, published in the journal *Neuroscience*, adds new evidence to the theory that non-steroidal anti-inflammatory drugs such as ibuprofen and aspirin may prevent this brain disease...

The team mixed a chemical marker that highlights plaque with diseased human brain tissue (in a test tube). They then added naproxen or ibuprofen, painkillers often used to treat arthritis pain.

...the researchers found the drugs melted away some of the plaque.

...The findings need to be confirmed with human studies... Will take years...

...warns against popping these drugs, even over-the-counter ibuprofen, in hopes of staving off dementia. These drugs can increase the risk of stomach bleeding, a problem that can be hazardous for older people.

Reference to *Beyond Aspirin*, Chapter 18 (page 194 of this book). An alternative, the herb Gotu Kola can be used without the side effects of the ibuprofen or aspirin.

May 12, 2003

dream...

A little girl, dark curly hair. Eyes knowing. Already quite a personality. She's waiting for her body to grow big enough to be born.

Quite content and safe.

Our soon to be new grandchild.
Is she my mother's soul ready to try again?
Would I lose her guidance if she was?
If you can "come around" again are you gone from those who feel you?

Only time on "earth" appears to be finite. Life has no time.
So, yes, Mama, you can "be her" and still be infinite at the same "time."
I would not lose your guidance...

May 2003

My sister and I share back to back appointments with
Dr. Brooks, Neurologist, at the University clinic. I am very
excited to go, because I have been feeling so much better.
My sister, also, has felt at least a stability.

The tests turn out well, some increase in strength, although
not 100% as there is also some decline. But the improvements seem to overpower the decline. I am confident we
will have a good report.

I state my positive attitude, my feeling of "survivor." Maybe
it is because of my new found "strength," or attitude; but
Dr. Brooks is finally upfront with us. He warns us "to keep it
all in perspective." We have found environmental factors,
not cures. The cure may be left to the next generation. It
will fall into the hands of genetics. Clearly our illness is
genetic, and we don't know what environmental factors are
affecting this, but we cannot focus on just one.

It is extremely important for us to be involved in the DNA
aspects and so it is Dr. Brooks' job to make sure the raw
data is down, to document, so the genetic studies can
continue. They may not figure it out in our lifetime, but what
we do now is crucial for other generations. Looking at the
documents 10 to 20 years from now they may hold a
different answer with a bigger picture.

After years of feeling lost and "unreal," I come into an
appointment feeling optimistic and proud of the advances

I've made, stronger in mind. Finally we are being talked to as an equal, a partnership. Another major step - finally being up front with our family.

It took all these years to be put into the right "slot." You would think I should be devastated. I am not. Being "unreal" is fake and leads to limbo. "Real" can be fought, analyzed, researched. I cannot fix what I don't know is broken. I can fix what I know is broken.
I already have - I am on my way.

For us, it never has been about quantity of life, but, quality of life. Life will have limitations, but I can love...
Why was being "real" so important?

1   The biggest chance for fighting the genetic factor comes from early detection. It took +15 years for mine to be recognized after extreme losses and a great loss in quality of life.
My sister was found at the very first, early sign. She has less loss and a higher quality of life.

2   It is much easier to research what is real and not a phantom illness. I never knew which direction I should be going. That is not all bad, perhaps I kept a broader picture.

3   Peace of mind.
I am not "crazy."
I am intelligent.
I am me...

May 14, 2003
This book has been the next step in my healing.
By organizing all the fragments into pieces and the pieces
into the puzzle, I am becoming whole, the next step of many
beyond survival.
I have learned how to survive.
Now I have to relearn how to live.

My older brother and I spent the day together in Madison, at
the Wisconsin Alzheimer's Registry for Research: Children of
parents with proven Alzheimer's. It was to obtain a base
line for further statistical research and to be given the
opportunity to participate in other studies.

One study of great interest to me was a functional brain
imaging using an MRI. I have had several MRI's, but during
this one they ask you questions to see how your brain
functions, or if there is any damage noted.

After many days of phone tag I speak with the study
co-coordinator of the research. I answer questions and
questions. In the end, I am rejected - my medicines are too
strong.
I am too far along to be a participant.

June 2003   Mom

I'm at our store, bringing in supper, when I'm handed the phone. "I thought I was OK before, but now I'm not."

It's Mom, my Mother-in law. "OK, I'll be right there." I'm not prepared for the sight before me when I arrive. I find her sitting on a dining room chair, phone in hand. She's black and blue from the top of her head to the bottom of her neck. Her right eye is swollen and purple. I'm afraid for her sight, a paper towel is wrapped around her arm. She's on the phone to a friend, asking about tomorrow's plans. I take the phone and tell her I'll call her back, I have to get Mom to the hospital.

She is a dynamic 84 years young. Upset this year that she found herself sitting through her favorite "soaps" instead of breaking to vacuum during the commercials! Independent, with a full schedule of events throughout the week. The social leader in her group. Working out at the "club" twice a week. And still maintaining an at home accounting business-although scaled back over the years. A thinker and keeper of ideas far beyond her time. Each year creating six works of art to give at Christmas.

Within hours I watch that all slip away. She tries to read the clock-the numbers loosing value. Her words become garbled-making no sense.

"Where am I? What's wrong?"

Fear...

Isolation....

Mom

She has a fractured skull, with a brain bruise, a broken collar bone in two places, and a sprained ankle. Her brain is not processing the information. We are told the brain is swelling. Inflammation. I know that word!

The doctors have no answers, only to watch, and wait. I know aromatherapy will not hurt her. In her room I spray a simple aromatherapy of rose water and jasmine in a blend. I bring in a gentle lotion of relaxing and anti-inflammation oils to use in her daily care. And the niceties of home, her pillow and favorite down throw. Anything that can keep her connected. The brain swelling stops before the critical point is reached, although a lot of damage has already occurred. The nurses comment on how well she's doing. How nice she and her room smell. She has to start over, to relearn what she no longer remembers.

After the four weeks in the hospital on the rehab floor, we have made a home for her in our home. We see so much of the same mental problems that I had experienced. Our daughter is able to match times in my life to hers. There is quite the understanding of what has happened, how she feels, what she is experiencing. Today when asked how she feels in our home, she said "protected." She quickly decides she will have nothing to do with anything that looks "handicapped." She fights to learn how to walk about the house unaided, and without a walker. It takes her less than a week.

Mom

We have arranged her clothes on open shelving in her room so she can see what she has, similar to how I have mine. She likes the set-up. It reduces a lot of stress. In two more weeks she has mastered the phone—to call her friends and family. Answering the phone is still a big hurdle.

August 5   Mom

Today we added in Omega 3, increased Calcium and an Eyebright blend to the Gotu Kola started in July.

This afternoon we watched Kirk Douglas on Oprah. His fight and determination to get back what he could from his stroke seven years ago, and to stay in the public eye is so encouraging to any one who has had any brain injury. He has found his family and their support. Wow, seven years! We are just starting.

August 7   Mom

Tonight as we talked she said *"I know it can't be like this, but sometimes my brain feels like before the accident and it is working. And everything is OK. I know that isn't right. And then it all goes away and it doesn't work. And I don't know my words again."*

I repeat it back to make sure I understood. And yes, for a short time - minutes only, she feels like she did before the accident. This is so great! I did not expect this just nine weeks after her injury. We are on the right road!

We just don't know how long this road will be!

But it is the right road!

Mom   **The steps we are taking are:**

Step 1   Nutrition

Protein and more protein "*In normal people protein contributes about 10 to 15 % of the energy required for normal body metabolism. In head-injured patients, 160 to 240% increases in protein administration were needed to obtain the same level of systemic metabolic activity, where nitrogen was used as the measure of balance.*"   BRAIN REPAIR, Chapter 9 (See Chapter III, pg 48)

There were a couple days in a row where protein was low in the meals, on the third day, she was talking incoherently unable to find the right words.

Step 2 Sleep like a baby

Newspaper: The Post-Crescent Tuesday, Aug 19, 2003

Researcher's brain booster: Sleep on it

They are finding in research trials that catching a nap might just be the best strategy for learning new motor and visual skills such as playing a musical instrument, hitting a golf ball straight or spotting birds in the woods. It turns out a 30 to 60 minute nap can improve motor-skill development by allowing the brain to process and store the newly learned information while the body is resting. The hypothesis is that your brain reaches a saturation point of neural connections when learning a new skill. This overload adversely affects the brain's performance as the day unfolds, rather than causing it to falter because of general body fatigue. "Power naps" improve alertness, mood, productivity and capability of learning new things.

Mom

Step 3 Supplements

Vitamin E An antioxidant

Omega 3 The right kind of fat for the brain. The brain itself is composed largely of fat. Each neuron is approximately 60 percent fat. For the improvement of cell membrane fluidity and improves nerve conduction within the optic nerve.

Aspirin, 81 mg A preventative.

Gotu Kola We first try Ginkgo Biloba, a more common herb for the brain. I watch for any reaction - she develops a headache just like my husband, her son. We switch to Gotu Kola a less known brain herb, but one that works extremely well. Her "searching for words" begins to diminish as Gotu Kola aids in the processing center of the brain.

Multi Vitamin

Eyebright complex The eyes have a separate blood-barrier. This complex is for increased health of the eyes and optic system.

Aromatherapy For relaxation and healing; a stress reducer.

Topical application Because the skin is the largest organ of the body, beneficial herbs/oils can be absorbed directly into the blood system. I use this method for anti-inflammatory herbs like rosemary, ginger, green tea, etc.

Step 4 Supportive environment with sensory and cognitive stimulation in a meaningful setting. (Responding to her great grandchildren, going out with her family and friends.)

August 2003

Our 4 year old grandson has spent the last year creating "machines." He started with large cardboard blocks and would make a new machine that would sit on the floor of his bedroom for a couple of days. He would explain its job to each of us and then create a new one. They not only became more elaborate with buttons and switches, but also more exotic. The first ones had general purposes like "garbage eater" and "dinosaur digger." Later they had jobs for only little boys imaginations like "of-noe-din-orator." The machines entered his drawings and we talked of blueprints. And then the machines expanded into our household, made with whatever parts he could find. He has probably made over a hundred machines, each with its own purpose, and a different design.

His great-grandmother, whom he is very close to, is still having a lot of memory/processing problems since her accident. He has picked up on this. It has been very hard on him because he doesn't understand how she can be so different in only a short time.

His last three machines have been "memory machines." He made one life-size for himself, crawled through it, and announced, "This one is so you will always have memory of this house." Today he made one with the help of Great-grandmother - she even had to help operate it! She had to listen very carefully and follow his directions so as not to disappoint him.
It was a memory machine for remembering Zebras.

August 5, 2003

**A letter from the Wisconsin Alzheimer's Institute,
University of Wisconsin, Madison**

I am writing to thank you for your participation in the
Wisconsin Registry for Alzheimer's Prevention (WRAP) and to
provide you with a project update and a summary of the results
so far. Currently, we have over 300 persons enrolled in WRAP.
We also have a list of about 70 interested persons who are
eligible for testing and enrollment. Our goal is to reach a total
enrollment of 500 adult children within the next two years.

We recently completed an analysis of the baseline data. The
average age of a WRAP participant is 53, 71% of you are
women, 77% are married and 68% are employed full-time.
You are a highly educated group with an average of 16 years of
education. This high level of education is reflected in the
testing results. Many of you commented that the neuropsychological testing overwhelmed you. Do not worry! The tests
are designed to challenge your abilities, and everyone should
expect to miss questions. This "intellectual challenge" is
necessary if we are to identify changes in cognitive function in
the future. You will be interested to know that the average IQ
is 113 which is phenomenal. This is far above average (100)
and might suggest that on average, WRAP participants may be
at a lower risk of developing Alzheimer's symptoms than the
general population. The research question is whether future
testing will indicate declines in cognition in certain persons and
whether that decline can be slowed or stopped.

We have expanded enrollment in WRAP. Enrollment in WRAP was initially restricted to the children of persons who were diagnosed with Alzheimer's disease at the University. This has now changed, and enrollment in WRAP is possible for any adult child who is able to provide outside medical records that document the diagnosis of Alzheimer's disease in their parent. Verification of the diagnosis is a time-consuming process, but is critically important to ensure the scientific integrity of WRAP.

We have created a newsletter entitled *Alzheimer's Update* that will be mailed to you at least twice a year. The purpose of the newsletter is to provide you with an update on WRAP and an update on the latest information about Alzheimer's research. If you are interested in a particular subject and if it might be of interest to a larger audience, we will try to include it in the newsletter. Send a letter or call.

I want to thank you again for participating. As I have told some of you, the original concept for WRAP was my wife's idea. Her mother recently died of Alzheimer's disease. I think all of us are concerned about ourselves and our children in the future. You are doing your job, and now it is our responsibility to develop the resources that will allow us to do the kind of world-class research that will make a difference.
Sincerely,

Mark A. Sager, M.D. Professor of Medicine
Director, Wisconsin Alzheimer's Institute

August 25, 2003
You can feel the door open between the worlds at birth and at death. Our Maclean Rose, born today, she is who we saw in our dreams, she is not a stranger, her dark hair - yet to grow long enough to curl. She reaches - already reaching for the life she wants to live.

I am laying in bed for a nap with Max, now 4 years old. Maclean Rose was born this morning. A very clear "Chris" echoes through the room. I know there is no one "here" to call my name. The voice is not immediately recognizable to me, but I know it has come through the "door."
I feel secure and unafraid.
I later recognize the voice as a chorus of voices,
not one single voice....
A chorus of voices...
Of all my guides

September 2003
Our daughter returns from a doctor appointment for Maclean. The pediatrician takes down the family health information. Since our daughter is nursing the pediatrician wants her to be sure to take Vitamin E, Folic acid, Omega 3's and baby aspirin supplements for the baby's protection. We now have validation of the nutritional benefits in all four generations.
I am pleased. Perhaps this now will stop with me.

September 18, 2003

Today is my 55th birthday.

Our house is full today. We have a daughter who has just given birth, a newborn, a 4 year old preschooler, and their great-grandmother.

I now have the strength to share my life with them.

What a birthday blessing - Thank you, Mama, for showing me the way.

My daughter comes down from an upstairs nap. "Mom, I have something very important for you to put into your book. I have a message from Grandma (your mother), I felt her so close. It is so real!"

Today you have under one roof to care for
a newborn, a 4 year old, a daughter, and a Mother-in-law.
And you are strong enough to handle it.

She didn't know I too shared the same thoughts that day...

I am so happy that we are so connected... that she, too, can share in the circle of life.

A validation.

November 7, 2003

A letter from University of Washington Alzheimer's Disease Research Center

Thank you for your ongoing interest in our research on Alzheimer's Disease and other dementias. The University of Washington Alzheimer's Disease Research Center is now in its 18th year of research, with continued support from the National Institutes of Health. Our genetic studies have screened more than 1500 families with Alzheimer's Disease or other dementias. Family history information, clinical records, blood samples, skin biopsies and autopsy findings from these families provide the basis for our scientific projects. This represents one of the largest collections in the world of information and material on familial Alzheimer's Disease and other dementias.

Our genetic studies have focused on early onset familial Alzheimer's Disease (before age 65), late onset familial Alzheimer's Disease (after age 65) and other dementias, such as frontotemporal dementia (sometimes called Pick's Disease) and Lewy Body disease (a combination of Alzheimer's Disease and Parkinson's Disease). We have a continuing interest in Alzheimer's Disease occurring in families whose background is German from Russia. We have been successful in helping to identify two genes, Presenilin 1 and Presenilin 2, which are responsible for some early onset familial Alzheimer's Disease, and one gene, tau, that is responsible for some familial frontotemporal dementia. These discoveries have provided important clues to understanding the biochemical changes that occur in the brain with Alzheimer's Disease and frontotemporal dementia and have offered research new opportunities for developing medications to treat AD.

The cause of late onset familial Alzheimer's Disease remains unknown. A major focus of our current research is to better understand genetic factors in late onset familial Alzheimer's Disease. Researchers think there are several genes contributing to late onset Alzheimer's Disease. We are collaborating with 15 other Alzheimer's Disease Research Centers on a new national project, the Late Onset Alzheimer's Disease (LOAD) Study. The LOAD Study is developing a National Cell Repository for Alzheimer's Disease, where information and material can be shared among qualified researchers. Families included in the LOAD study have two or more brothers or sisters living with late onset Alzheimer's Disease. We believe that this combined effort will help identify the genes involved in late onset familial Alzheimer's Disease.

Accurate, updated family history information is critical to our research. If there have been changes in your family, please notify us. As we review our records on families involved in our research, we may be calling you to update the family history information.

Alzheimer's Disease and other dementias present great challenges for patients, for families and for researchers. With your help, we have made significant progress in understanding Alzheimer's Disease and frontotemporal dementia, which we believe will lead us toward more effective treatment and prevention. We greatly appreciate your involvement in this research, and we look forward to continuing to work together on these projects. If you have any questions or concerns, please contact us.

Sincerely,

Thomas D. Bird, M.D.
Neurologist, Geriatric Research Center
VA Puget Sound Health Care System
Professor, Neurology and Medical Genetics
University of Washington School of Medicine

Ellen (Nemens) Steinbart, R.N., M.A.
Malia Rumbaugh, M.S., C.G.C.
Alzheimer's Disease Research Center
University of Washington
VA Puget Sound Health Care System

December 2003

dream….

Like white clouds wisping by, I am surrounded by
energy. Strong enough to lift, it floats me up and down
on a bed of soft down. It feels strong, yet comforting.
I use all my senses to "feel it"…
it is euphoria…
my senses take me deeper…
it is healing….
it is health…
I "float" in contentment.
We are standing still, my daughter next to me.
Cows are rushing towards us… they look out of control…
a stampede… my childhood fear…
Should we run? Should we stop the dream?
"No. Watch… the cows will stop." I say.
And so they do, right next to me. I reach out
and pet a slippery, wet, black nose.
All is safe.

I relate this dream to my daughter the next day. I am
excited about the healing feeling.
She adds, "Yes, but look at the rest, you not only faced the
danger/fear, but you were in control. You 'handled' it."
Yes…
I am once again living.

My Child, The Farm Responds
When the words to this poem were put down on paper,
I thought it was being written for my children - the lessons I
wanted them to remember, that I may not always be able
to say.

I now realize that "My Child" is me and these are the
lessons I needed to relearn.
The words were not from me, but through me.

My Child
The Farm Responds

My Child
Feel the children of the farm,
Those who have come before you.
Know their mysteries of life past,
Walk in their steps,
Feel what they have felt,
Love what they have loved.

Learn of a future promised to you,
For this is the road of your growth.
Follow with confidence,
Pass it on to yours…
With love

My Child
Find the last of a great tree
Ancient I am.
Cut with a mighty hand,
Stump and log head high.
Among the tall grasses
I lay with pride.

Crawl upon my back and play.
Feel my hidden strength directing you forward.
I have felt when there was not yet a child.
In my veins ran earth's energy
Even now they are full.

Explore in safety.
Look unto your promised future.
Pluck splinters of wood from my stump
Using them as instruments of your imagination.
Become a doctor or nurse with patients,
A sailor with ship's mates playing "I spy,"
Perhaps a cook, or a pilot flying high.
Find the value in knowledge.
Seek it always.

Know kindness, caring, patience and love.
As I once shared my great limbs
With the birds of the fields
And safely held their homes
Awaiting the rains without complaint.
Even now, my form gone, I am for all.
Learn…
Thereby continuing the flow of life

My Child
Duck under the fence and
Find the endless pastures.
Enter the vast "plains" where
Indians could come passing by,
Or buffalo -
Perhaps elephants led by Tarzan.
I hold the footprints of life past
Unique as they may be.

Crisscrossing paths share
Hidden clues to harmony.
I give you my treasures
Left by each that has passed through me.
Have respect for all that I hold.

Explore all paths,
Recognize the signs.
This will keep you on track
As I am endless to small feet.

Feel the sunshine upon my face.
My rumpled skin is
Shaped with respect and harmony.
Each particle of who I am
Has come from those about me.
Take them away and…
I grow no more

My Child
Approach the field of sentinels.
I give strength to the farm.
First to be planted, last to be harvested,
It is my corn that feeds the farm.

Walk among my many rows orderly in nature.
Feel my sheltering coolness,
A relief to little sunbathed heads.
My magnificent stalks nearly touch the clouds.

Do not lose sight of north and south
For then a maze I can quickly become
By towering over all.
Do not fear or run.

As I use my long leaves to know
that which surrounds me,
So too let the natural instinct within you
Guide you back on path.
For the key to your strength
Comes from….
Understanding the inner nature of all

My Child
Planted fresh each spring
I bring new life to the farm.
My fragile shoots form the grains of life.
Surround yourself in my new energy,
Find comfort in my sameness.

Green now –
Golden by the end of summer
To become a silken nest of straw
In the upper barn when harvested in fall.
Take time to relax in my softness.
As I multiply from one grain,
So too multiply the happiness of this world.

I am the sea of the land.
Sway with the winds
Like waves without water,
Feel the melodious rhythm.

Open your mind to the quiet within you
For there lies your oneness.
Smile…
I am bliss

My Child
I give shape to the farm
Connecting all that it holds.
Edged by fences,
Rutted by tractor tires and hooves,
Finely tuned by bicycle tires spun and
swirled,
I am the lane.

Open my gate that forms the beginning
Endless to little eyes.
Parts are dry sand with a rocky edge,
Others soft with moss in the shade of a tree.
A roller coaster of uneven land
Ever changing yet the same.
Feel secure in my form.

Experience the fields as they pass by.
Look close as you choose your way.
I am wide enough for change.
Some footprints follow the paths of others,
Others venture to higher ground.
Each forms my uniqueness
As long as you take the next step.

Rest under a tree
Buzzing with life as bees nest in its womb.
See where you have been.
By coming you have left a change in me.
Simple at the end I blend into a vast field.
Journey on…
I am your life

A New Beginning

My Child
Weary bones, Spent muscles
Heads seeking down pillows
Bedtime stories calm

Nighttime kisses shared
Patchworks of love snugly protect
Dreams await opening

Growing bodies sprout
Sleeping babies rejuvenate Moms
Hooting owls serenade

Tooth fairies making rounds
Santa's elves gathering wishes
Moon's energies abound

Dewdrops capture day's heat
Three o'clock stillness explodes
Minds free, Bodies rest

Problems presented
Clues float quickly by
Solutions proposed

Minds rest, Bodies stir
Moon's energy abates
Birds chatter in seasonal patterns

Day breaks in rhythm
A new beginning...
For all

I am learning to live with limitations.

I am learning to use all my senses in finding my life and the ability to live... Hearing, seeing, smell, taste, and touch are but the beginning.
Add in instinct, coincidences, déjà vu and intuition.
Along with bliss, humming, and healing dreams.

If I feel stressful, I "hum." On the way to an appointment, I found myself becoming very anxious to the point of becoming nauseous. I knew I had no way to cancel the appointment, so I remembered to hum. I started to hum along to the songs on the radio, and within a couple of songs the stress was gone, and I was relaxed!
Cortisol under control!

I was able to stop additional damage to my body. And that is my goal.

If the disease sneaks away parts of me, I find I have other parts to replace them. In re-teaching myself to cook, I find I am now cooking by "hearing." My fried egg makes a certain sound as it cooks and I can tell if I forgot to turn down the burner by the sound.

"Simple" is how I will live and relearn. I am in tune with whatever signals I can feel from my body and the universe around me.

THE PIECES TO THE PUZZLE ARE COMING TOGETHER:

- Emotional Support
  - Family
  - Understanding Doctors
  - Friends and Strangers
- Balance
  - Mind
  - Body
  - Spirit
- Hope
  - Healing Intelligence
- Endorphins
  - Laughter
  - Touch
  - Massage
  - Yoga / QiGong / Reiki
- Meditation
  - Bliss
  - Humming - Om
  - Prayer
- Creativity
  - Thinking
  - Reading
  - Arts
- Rest / Sleep

- Nutrition
  - Protein
  - Complex Carbo's
  - Omega 3 Fats
  - Vitamins
  - Minerals
  - Anti-oxidants
- Anti-MSG
- Anti-Aspartate
- Anti-Inflammation
- Herbs
  - Supplements
  - Herbal Baths
  - Topical
- Medications
- Psyche
  - Healing Dreams
  - Coincidence
  - Déjà Vu
  - Intuition
- Energy
  - Universal
  - Mind/Body/Heart
  - Spiritual

HEALING LOVE

January 1, 2004 The *Post-Crescent* Newspaper

Troubles Spell Doom for Lab at Medical School

Madison - The University of Wisconsin Medical School
has closed a neurology laboratory....motor/muscle testing...

My Response

As a family, who has had three generations as patients of Dr. Brooks at the UW Medical School neurology clinic, we have had first hand experiences with the motor/muscle testing from its inception, sometimes every three months.

You may wonder what these tests are able to tell us and how important are they?

Imagine this: One day you see your shoe laying on the floor upside down. When you pick it up you notice that one whole side of the sole is worn thin, like you must have been unconsciously dragging your foot. Why? Or you reach to turn over a glass in the cupboard and your hand won't grasp the glass. Why? Or you are walking down the aisle in a store and you find you are suddenly tipping to the right. You catch yourself this time. Why? Or you are getting up off the couch only to fall back down. Why? Slowly, very slowly, changes are occurring. Why? The changes continue, taking every part of your life away. Who will listen? Who has the answer? How can anyone measure these progressive, subtle changes? Who will be able to tell us the "why"?

The UW neurology clinic was and is at the cutting edge of finding these answers. I have been to several neurologists over the years, and no one else has tested for or seen the small, but very significant changes that were occurring. I was more than once told it was all in "my head." Until it had taken the very "me" away. With the testing at the UW neurology clinic we are able to see the progression; or, when trying different medications, the stabilization; or, in really good situations, some reversal of the disease. Again, in most of the neurological diseases the changes are subtle and the measurements need to be precise.

We chose Dr. Brooks and the UW Medical School neurology clinic in order to be a part of the excellent research and the positive results from this research. There were no cures for these neurological diseases when the testing began. The testing is performed in a highly professional manner, with complete patient consent throughout each step of the testing. Never did I ever feel in danger. We were not once left alone with a student or lab worker tester.

By removing these tests, **someone** thinks our lives will be safer. Let me tell you, you have just set mine, and hundreds of others, death dates. It has taken over **ten years,** just to find the what in my illness, the same illness that took our mother's life.

Because of the research done with me, it only took **three months** to find it and less than a year to stabilize it in my sister. With the cancellation of the testing, neither of us will have the advantage of early detection of any future changes in progression. Because of the testing, my children have a baseline, but with the cancellation of the testing, they no longer will have their chance for early diagnosis.

How can any person in clear conscience, doom hundreds of people, plus multiple generations to come, to a life less than what it could be? How can any person in clear conscience go backward in research? I can only guess it is the money. How do you, decide for me if I have been "inconvenienced and put at risk" without even asking me? And how do you know what my life has been and now will be because of your actions!!

My medications may be short term. When I once again, with any progression of my disease not caught early do to lack of testing, am no longer able to hold my grandchildren, what do I say to them? And if they are stricken, how do I tell my children and my grandchildren that "if only...."

We were never inconvenienced, put at risk, or had our *patient's rights* compromised by Dr. Brooks or the muscle/motor laboratory. However, we have been inconvenienced, put at risk, and have had our *patient's rights* compromised by those that made the decision to close this muscle/motor laboratory.

Thank you

March 2004

It has been over a year since my last appointment with
Dr. Cooper at the Memory Center in Oshkosh. I am taken into
a room to be given the memory tests. Last year I did pretty
well. Although I do seem to be learning most of the answers,
you cannot learn the list of words they use in the "repeat
these words back to me" section because they use different
words each time. I am given 5 different tests. I do very well.
The lady giving me the test is amazed. This seldom happens
at a memory clinic. We talk a bit. She is from the Alzheimer's
Association and filling in for the testing. I explain my
nutritional regimen. She gives me a brochure for the
upcoming statewide Alzheimer's Conference in Madison,
Wisconsin. "Maybe you'll want to go."

Dr. Cooper is thrilled with my testing, "What have you been
doing? The tests are perfect - 'scareingly' perfect. This
aggressive approach of the anti-inflammatory herbs, along
with the Omega 3's is a step beyond the researchers, but it
makes sense... unbelievable results... but it makes sense.
Keep up the good job!"

It's been a year and a half that I have been using the anti-
inflammatory bath teas, along with the Omega 3's, Vitamin E,
and the herb regimen; combined with the nutrition,
medicines, stress reduction and exercise that was already in
place. I go home with a heightened sense of validity.

I chose *Research-Seek,* 14 years ago, never expecting the
level of guidance I would receive.

Dr. Cooper's research has included the importance of the ratio of Omega 3 and Omega 6 essential fatty acids. Essential fatty acids must be provided by dietary sources. (Olive oil, flaxseed, walnuts, leaf plants, fish, seaweed, seafood are Omega 3's. Corn oil, safflower oil, meats are Omega 6's.) I had thought that the main purpose for the essential fatty acids was as a nutritional source for the brain, the basis for cell membranes and the creation of hormones. If we eat the correct fatty acids, our cellular membranes are strong, flexible, and discriminating. The brain neurons are composed of 60% fat.

But Dr. Cooper's work points out that Omega 3's and 6's also control inflammation at the cellular level. Omega 3's are anti-inflammatory, and Omega 6's are pro-inflammatory. A diet balanced with low Omega 6's and adequate Omega 3's, and high in antioxidants should protect neuronal cell membranes from the initial damage of lipid oxidation and the destructive cascade of inflammation and brain lesions. The possibility exists that the development and progression of Alzheimer's Disease may be slowed or arrested with an aggressive intervention.

Oxidation results from excess inflammation, causing cellular membranes to break down, releasing toxins that further damage cells, causing more inflammation. If the body cannot keep up with the resulting damage and release of toxins, a cascade of more inflammation, more oxidation, more cell death begins.

MY LEVELS OF INTERVENTION

PLAQUE ◄─────► Step 1. Gotu Kola Eliminates PLAQUE

Tooth decay/gum disease from Plaque on teeth.

Stroke/heart disease from Arterial Plaque.

Alzheimer's disease from Amyloid Plaque.

(Note: Neurofibrillary tangles have been found in the

brain, liver, pancreas, ovary, testes and thyroid)

BRAIN INJURY, ENVIRONMENT, CHEMICALS, STRESS,

EXCESS EXCITOTOXINS (AMINO ACIDS) ◄─────► Step 2.

Reduce SAFETY risk factors, Control STRESS, Reduce

use of TOXINS, Glutamate (MSG), Aspartame

(NutraSweet©), and L Cysteine (in bread).

Add Omega 3's, Herbs, Vitamins, Minerals

Brain injury can start the inflammation process.

Humming, meditation, and energy work remove

stress, keep Cortisol under control.

Excess excitatory amino acids (glutamate, aspartate,

cysteine) cause destruction of brain cells,

which causes inflammation.

INFLAMMATION ◄─────► Step 3. Anti-inflammatory Herbs

Decrease INFLAMMATION

The COX-2 inflammatory response to plaque is out of

balance with the actual threat of the plaque.

Inflamed neurofibrillary tangles/plaque form lesions.

Inflammation becomes out of control.

FREE RADICALS OF OXYGEN ◄─────► Step 4. Anti-oxidents

Omega 3's, Herbs, Vitamins, Minerals are FREE

RADICAL SCAVENGERS eliminating oxidants.

A result of unchecked inflammation = oxidation = cell

death = release of toxins = more inflammation ==='s

May 2004

Where am I at now?

The advantage to supplementing with herbs is that you can adjust with your needs. Having a bad week, you can adjust with a bit more. Weather is good, getting lots of rest, you can adjust down. And change herbs to match symptoms.

My pharmacological drugs at this time are: Amantadine, Eldepryl/Selegiline, Atenolol, Plavix, and Zincate. I have been able to decrease the dosage since the start of the herbal anti-inflammatory regimen on some of these.

The nutrition supplements include multi-vitamin (3 times the regular dosage), additional vitamin E and Omega 3's.

My herbal regimen includes Ginkgo Biloba, Gotu Kola, Schizandra, Damiana, White Willow, Red Raspberry, Red Clover, and Passion Flower. These are supplemented with a bath soak of tea made from Green Tea, Rosemary, Ginger, Lemon Balm and Gotu Kola three to four times a week as an aid for inflammation. I alternate this with Green Heart's Auntie's Anti, a topical blend of anti-inflammation oils. I am also careful to use face and hair products with Rosemary or other anti-inflammation herbs.

Increase in protein, moderate complex carbohydrates, no MSG, or MSG suspected foods, no artificial sweeteners, and using organic or home grown foods are my dietary goals.

Tuning into the healing energy. And a good dose of laughter!

May 2, 2004

Watch for the coincidences in life......

My sister and I are sitting in the back of "the grand ball-room" having arrived late to the opening speaker at the Wisconsin State Alzheimer's Conference. During the mid-point break, I offer to watch the chairs for the women a row ahead. After a few minutes one of the ladies introduces herself and we exchange information. They are here be-cause her husband is suffering from a form of dementia, but not Alzheimer's. I tell her of myself, and she wants all the information on my Eastern/Western blended approach.

After listening to the opening speaker, my sister and I check out the books being sold by the Alzheimer's Association. I inquire as to how the books were chosen. My sister tells them that I have a book in the works. They add encouraging remarks and more questions. They tell me I must attend the workshop entitled "The Voices of Alzheimer's Disease" to be presented on Monday by several people diagnosed with early-stage Alzheimer's.

Because of the continued inquiring, my sister suggests that we put together a quick flyer to hand out to people when they ask. It is obvious that any information on any type of success is sought. I work on the flyer that night and in the morning we run off copies at a copy shop.

It is my plan to talk with the moderator of the early stage group before they begin, but, upon arriving I see she is needed to encourage and settle her panel of speakers. I listen to their remarks through the program and feel just as they have felt. I am a part of them. I'm not sure that I will speak out. In closing, she asks her panel for their last remarks. A gentle man states he has two ideas: 1) that he is lucky. Because he is into his seventies and that it would have been much worse for him if he had Early Onset Alzheimer's and he was younger. 2) "If we could only stay put," he wishes for a way not to get worse.

Questions from the audience. There sit those coincidences. I raise my hand, and take a deep breath. I tell them I am one of those you spoke of who is working through the early onset form. I have been where they are. (My mind is telling me the words are not flowing out very well. The ideas are getting stuck in my head. There is so much more I want to say.) I rattle on a very little more. Letting them know that I have had success incorporating herbs and Eastern medicine along with the usual drugs. I have a handout for anyone who is interested. Not to take away from the wonderful presentation they have just completed. I quickly sit. Applause fills the room. People are reaching from all directions for the flyer. I am stunned. The applause was for me!
Encouragement!

I hand out more flyers and answer more questions after the program. I am asked to attend an early onset support group near our home. I will go.

My sister was attending a workshop on pharmacological interventions while I was in the panel group lecture. She is very excited because the doctor giving the lecture has agreed to talk with us for a bit. He does not have much new insight into our mother's or our processes. But it is OK. My sister is learning much more about the disease and will now understand more of what I have been trying to say.

We bump into the Alzheimer's Association Executive Director of the South Central Chapter before we leave. He was also in the room for "The Voices of Alzheimer's Disease." He states that my words to the group in the few, short, stated paragraphs let everyone both feel where I have been and know how I have come back.

Wow! I didn't think I had done a very good job!
He encourages my sister and me to continue to speak out and to talk personally to as many researchers as possible.

We both are very exhausted at the end of the day. But the day is not over. My sister's family is in the process of moving to a newer home. She gets word that the people who are going to wax the wood floors in the old house have moved their date to tomorrow. After a nice dinner we go over to clear the floors. This was bad timing for her to have attended a conference, but within a couple hours we are able to get all the floors ready. I think we had a bit of "outside" help. The whole conference has been like that. "Give of yourself and you are given back thrice."

On the last day, I question some, and speak out a bit more (I write down my thoughts so I sound a bit more together) and am asked to give out a few more flyers. I approach several researchers, but am pretty much "shot down." Until the last session of the conference. The speaker is from the University of Wisconsin, Madison, Memory Research Program and Geriatric Research and Clinic. He speaks on current research, but feels most everything has been said over the course of the three days. His personality is the greatest. Everyone encourages him, just to talk. He perfectly describes one part of Mama's disease, Balint's Syndrome, that we never understood.

We question whether a person afflicted with Alzheimer's can have multiple types. And yes, there are a great percentage of people who will fit into that scenario of mixes.
It is like the puzzle pieces are fitting together.

In the question period there is a man who states that we have heard a lot of information, can the doctor or anyone else put it into words a lay person can understand....
Please... Please... Please...

We pass him a flyer, and he is most thankful. But his pleading will stay with me a long time.

My sister and I approach the doctor. I welcome him to Wisconsin because I know he has come from Washington

State and he studied with Dr. Bird. I explain that our family line has been picked up for genetic studies through Dr. Bird.

He accepts our flyer and scans over it right then. "Yes, yes, yes." He also reads over a copy of Mama's autopsy report. I have my sister ask if he will accept her as a patient, he wants both of us. I tease him and ask what will he do for us. "No, no. I'm afraid it will be what I will learn from you." He states we are to see him ASAP.

This conference took a lot to attend, both emotionally and logistically. I felt our mother and all my guides surrounding me and guiding me through these days, "thick like pudding." I smile for days after. I know what I have achieved is real.... I have accepted the responsibility to pass on the information to help others. No one addresses the "big" picture. They mostly speak of "magic pills" but as researchers that is their direction. I can show the whole picture and not offend anyone.

Perhaps by sharing, it will help keep one more family intact.

A look at the basis of the FDA approved drugs:

The first class of drugs for Alzheimer's is based on the neurotransmitter acetylcholine. The primary carrier of thought and memory. It is believed that the levels of acetylcholine are low due to damage or death of cells. In order to increase the available amount of acetylcholine, these drugs inhibit the break down of acetylcholine.

> donepezil (Aricept)
> rivastigmine (Exelon)
> galantamine (Reminyl)

Naturally:

Acetylcholine is made from the nutrient choline in our bodies.

* Choline is present in high amounts in lecithin which also helps the body to digest and transport fat. It also keeps cholesterol soluble, and helps produce the bile acids that are made from cholesterol. (Perhaps possible links to fatty acid metabolism problems and cholesterol seen in Alzheimer's?)

* Lecithin is found in egg yolks, wheat germ, peanuts and peanut butter, liver, ham, soybeans and soybean oil, and whole wheat products.

* Supplements are inexpensive and nontoxic.

The second class of drugs for Alzheimer's is based on the over-stimulation of **excess glutamate**. It was first approved in Germany in 1982 for treatment of various neurological disorders (under Axura and Ebixa). Excess glutamate over-stimulates receptors allowing too much calcium into nerve cells, leading to disruption and death of cells. This drug acts by bonding to the cell receptors thus prohibiting the glutamate from bonding.

memantine (Namenda)

Naturally:

This information supports the findings reported in Chapter 10 *Excitotoxins, The Taste that Kills.*

* Elimination of MSG - under all of its names (monosodium glutamate), NutraSweet© (aspartate), and L Cysteine (in bread) from the diet would be step number one, thus helping to lower the toxic levels.

• Protection from the excitotoxins can be gained by incorporating vitamins E with C, K, D, A, and beta-carotene, minerals magnesium, chromium, zinc and selenium, plus a diet with adequate protein and complex carbohydrates for energy. Avoid low blood sugar levels and low oxygen (vascular delivery), as both compound the damage. Include nutrients such as Omega 3 fatty acids from flax seed oil or fish oils.

* Glutamate over-stimulation can cause cell mitochondrial DNA defect inheritance rather than the usual chromosomal DNA defect inheritance.

May 19, 2004

My sister, Mary Kay, and I have back-to-back appointments with Dr. Brooks at the UW Clinics.

Our sister, Rosann, and one of our brothers have also come down to Madison to participate in the Wisconsin Alzheimer's Registry Program for Children of a parent with confirmed Alzheimer's. To date there are over 450 participants. Our family will have six participants. It is important for further research.

This is the second time we have been able to co-ordinate our appointments together. Dr. Brooks comments that it is a growing trend in California - always knew we were on the cutting edge. He likes it because more information can be covered without having to repeat the basics. Also one person may pick up on a question the other had.

This is the first time in all my years of coming that the muscle/motor testing was not done. The University is "re-evaluating" the procedure to see if it is necessary. It is a great disappointment to us. Especially now, when we appear to have a breakthrough. Without the fine measure-ments it is very hard to tell if I have maintained, improved, or slipped backward. Without the measurements we don't know for sure if the herbs work in the same way as the prescription drugs. Without the measurements one year of documentation has been taken away.

I have typed up (as always) a two page report from my medical diary to give to Dr. Brooks. It is helpful for me, because it will take days for me to remember all that I want to discuss. Also, because of the stress of the day, I often find it hard to communicate my thoughts directly. He likes it because he can get a better picture of my health and also refer back to the notes later.

* I start with the date, my name and birth date.
* Listing the medications and supplements along with the dosage saves a lot of time for the nurses. If I have made any changes in the medications/supplements from my last visit, I state the reason for the change and/or a description of the new item. I include all nutritional supplements and herbs (including topical applications) so the full picture is very clear.
* Using my diary as a guide I continue with dates and events that occurred since my last appointment. This could be health, social, family, dreams, feelings, illnesses. Anything that has an impact on how I am doing.
* This is summarized with the answer to two questions: What is good (or better)? and What is worse (or still bad)?
* I then list any questions or comments I want to be sure to discuss.

I should state that, for me, my "diary" that I keep at home is a simple calendar with large blocks for the days. On this I keep my events and appointments, and also add my health and feelings, along with any changes in nutrition, supplements, and medications. It is a lot less formal than a book and works great. I can also mark off whole weeks with a feeling such as "legs hurt really bad" or "extra tired" or "felt great!"

Our appointment is very much more relaxed. There is a sharing of information among Dr. Brooks and our family members - with Dr. Brooks encouraging our questions and comments.

I relate that one of the concerns of Alzheimer's is that the brain does not produce enough of the so-called growth factors (biochemical compounds) that might help combat disease and injury. (See *Brain Repair 's Chapter 6*) I grew a Gotu Kola plant and saw that it is extremely prolific with not only, new plant shoots every four inches on long hanging vines, but also, hundreds of scattering seeds constantly falling. My question; Can plant growth factors be compatible with human growth factors? Dr. Brooks replies, "That's a very good question! And the answer is, yes. We have soy, and actually, alfalfa is the closest to humans."
(A plug for the *Green Juice* we see in the health food stores!)

One of our first cousins who has had by-pass heart surgery at a very early age has told us he has a hereditary factor for cholesterol with small sized LDL cells. Dr. Brooks is having us follow through to see if it runs in our family also.

We all await any results from the genetic studies. So far, there are no commercial DNA tests available so we are to be patient.

We are also to look into movement classes to reinforce the mind/body connection.

Dr. Brooks looks at me and states, "Taking what you have led us to... there is a new drug being designed that we may be able to use as a preventative for your family... It's not for sure... but it is looking good!"

That is so much better than even a year ago, when every-thing looked like generations away! My children... my siblings and cousins! Never to be on this journey!

There are a number of movement classes to choose from. Yoga, Tai Chi, dance, and Qi Gong are a few. Our daughter-in-law, Erika, has been studying medical Qi Gong. Not only is this a movement modality, but it is also an energy balancer. Qi (pronounced "chee") is the Chinese term for energy of a biological or universal nature. The nature of Qi and how it affects health comes from centuries of scientific observation of the laws of nature. The energy runs through the body on meridians enabeling the body and its organs to interrelate. Qi Gong is gentle and can be practiced by any-one. It works both physically and emotionally restoring the harmony of Qi thus increasing the body's healing power.

May 26, 2004

Newspaper article *The Post-Crescent*

Study Finds Aspirin Might Cut Risk of Breast Cancer

Associated Press

Chicago

Aspirin, the wonder drug that can help prevent heart attacks and strokes, also appears to reduce women's chances of developing the most common type of breast cancer, a study found.

The study appears in today's *Journal of the American Medical Association* and was led by researcher Mary Beth Terry and Dr. Alfred Neugut of Columbia University.

A regular intake of aspirin may lessen the cancer of breast cancer in women, especially for hormone-dependent cancers. Researchers theorize that the aspirin binds with and blocks COX-2 enzymes, catalysts in the synthesis of estrogen and the proliferation of tumor cells.

Another study released that supports the information in *Beyond Aspirin.*
Reference to chapter four of *Beyond Aspirin.*

In reviewing the information we received from the Wisconsin Alzheimer's Conference in May, I find an interesting paper, *Dementia Survival - A New Vision,* by Morris Friedell. Morris Friedell is a 63 year old retired professor who was diagnosed with Alzheimer's Disease in 1998. He wrote this paper outlining a 10 step rehabilitation program he uses to complete a task. He has presented at the International Alzheimer's Disease Conference. Some of his other papers include his use of music therapy, quality of life, and his journey. These can be accessed on his homepage (http://members.aol.com/MorrisFF/index.html). The full paper *Dementia Survival - A New Vision,* is at (http://members.aol.com/MorrisFF/vision.html).

In reviewing *Dementia Survival - A New Vision* I saw that my steps to relearning have followed his outline. I equated my learning to that of our infant grandson. Morris Friedell uses the approach of a young child and is based on the Montessori learning techniques This structured approach helps us "to go on living."

Dementia Survival - A New Vision

    Morris Friedell   March, 2001 (rev. December, 2003)

Section II of VI

    Ten Steps for Recovery of School-Age Competence

        (Instrumental Activities of Daily Living)

Theory: There is great potential for relearning problem-solving using new procedures involving a greater number of simpler steps.

* 1   HOPE: daring to believe it might be possible. After
        diagnosis, if we can recover much of our
        functioning for years, who are we then?
        We are in limbo.

* 2   WHY: we confront motivational obstacles. Why care,
        why try? Search for an answer in your deepest
        beliefs and memories.

* 3   ASSESSMENT: examine your life. What is your
        actual level of ability and disability? A good way to
        organize your "inventory" of abilities is go up
        through the years of childhood. Can you tie your
        shoes? Can you make a sandwich? Where do you start
        having trouble?

* 4   ACCEPTANCE: whatever you find in your inventory.
        It is important to work toward an attitude of
        unconditional acceptance.

* 5   REMEMBRANCE: what it was like to be a young
        child learning through play. Regain an attitude of
        wonder, exploration and engrossment. In play the
        child learns about self and world - verbal
        explanations are unnecessary.

        How do we manage if we can only think one
        thought at a time? Like a child, we learn through
        doing - through exploration and absorption. A
        sequence of "baby-steps" can lead one to amazing
        places. Repeat a simple activity until you feel
        assured. Then look for something more difficult to
        do, which stretches us but does not overwhelm us.

* 6   ENGAGEMENT: selecting a concrete problem and
       confronting it.
* 7   PERSEVERANCE: the willingness to walk through
       some moderate pain. It is normal to feel emotional pain
       in nakedly confronting one's deficits. It seems to be a
       law of human nature that change is sometimes difficult.
       Any distress needn't be severe or prolonged. Respite,
       support, and positive self-talk are invaluable.
* 8   VALIDATION: whatever the outcome of the project,
       take the time to reward and affirm yourself.
       Confront the implications of failure or success.
* 9   CONSOLIDATION: sufficient repetition is needed so
       that procedures can be well-habituated. These simple
       tasks can then be assembled into complex abilities.
*10   RESPITE: fatigue is onmipresent and cannot be
       taken for granted. Coping with fatigue improves
       opportunities for rehabilitation.

So - the ten steps are HOPE, WHY, ASSESSMENT,
ACCEPTANCE, REMEMBRANCE, ENGAGEMENT,
PERSEVERANCE, VALIDATION, CONSOLIDATION,
and RESPITE. The steps must be gone through many times,
considering the many activities comprising life, and they must
be repeated when the disease progresses. Yet each step builds
self-esteem. A person who is forced to slow down and simplify
may develop new creative and intuitive stengths. We need to
be able to process the challenges that face us.

In moving from victim to survivor our emotional sensistivity
can bring healing to ourselves and our family.

Our grandson loves to play with blocks....

I'm sitting on the floor next to our grandson (early two's at the time). In front of us is a pile of blocks ready to stack. He loves to play with blocks. He reaches and stacks the blocks one on one until the blocks topple over. He is ever so careful and can stack them almost as tall as he is, but they do topple over. I show him how to start with a strong base and then continue to build. He is fascinated with the results. Not only can he build taller, but he can build whole machines, buildings, and creatures.

So too, the books I have read work together to make a strong base, each one inter relating to the other.
All with the same basic theme.
Not "just the brain," but the whole body.
Not "just ME," but the whole universe.
I am able to build up from there,
To the end I am seeking
Healing... Living... Loving...

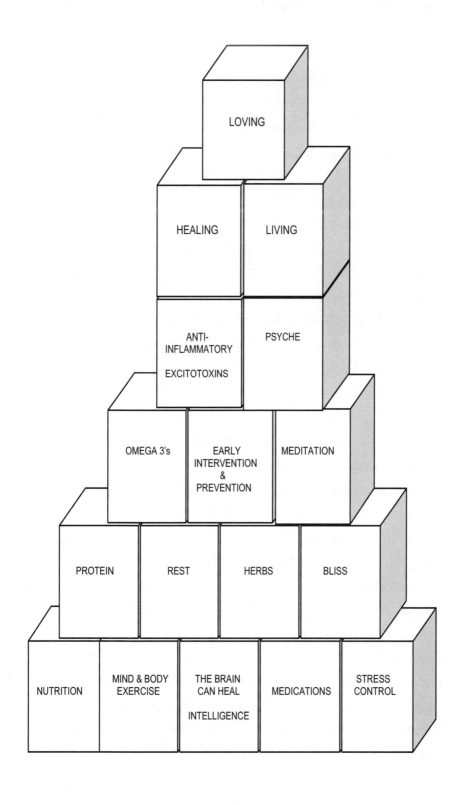

I am going to sneak in one more study which I have just found. Even as I ready the book for the printer, more and more information comes to light. My research will not end with this book. I am now in a "cascade of healing" where each little change for the better has a dramatic effect!

Blueberries have been under study since 2002 for their high antioxidant capacity. The low bush, wild, variety (Vaccinium angustifolium Aiton) have 16 different anthocyanin molecules which have been found to be neuroprotective. By testing on mice, it had previously been found that a diet rich in wild blueberries for six weeks dramatically protects neurons from stroke damage (Sweeney MI, Kalt W, MacKinnon SL, Ashby J, Gottschall-Pass KT.,*Nutr Neurosci. 2002 Dec; 5(6):427-31.*)

A new study shows that wild blueberry supplementation enhances signaling and prevents behavioral deficits in an Alzheimer's Disease model. The blueberry fed mice with Alzheimer's Disease actually preformed better than the non-inflicted controls in the Y-maze test. There is no known drug that can duplicate these results. (Joseph JA, Denisova NA, Arendash G, Gordon M, Diamond D, Shukitt-Hale B, Morgan D., *Nutr Neurosci. 2003 Jun;6(3):153-62.*)

Fresh or frozen wild blueberries are available, as is a concentrate (1 tablespoon equals one cup of wild blueberries), also look for jams and dried berries.
We drink juice everyday, so I will add wild blueberry juice to our regimen.

August 2004

My husband and I have always let our hands gently touch in passing. From our first date, 39 years ago, I let him know that I loved to touch and to be touched (being one of those sensitive, "touchy, feely, people"). So when this disease started, and I was ravaged with pain, touching was one of the physical expressions that was affected the most. I would "wince" in pain with a simple hug. But I always tried not to "flinch" because I wanted the affection, the sign of love and caring. I wanted to feel close. But he must have sensed it anyway.

It started about two weeks ago. Instead of just reaching for my hand, he now lays his hand on my back. The next time, he lays his hand on my back and gently moves it up and down. He continues to do this a couple of times before I realize what is happening. I look up at him and say, "Touching no longer hurts!" It had been a gradual loss. And now I realize how much it means for both of us. And how much we have missed it.

Touch. The nerve endings throughout my body must be healing. Inflammation under control. "Yes!" - to the herbal bath teas and the full regimen I have chosen!

Herbs

I was not alone on this journey, our family is close. Nor did I go "easily" onto this path of Eastern/Western healing. You might even say I resisted it for quite some time, until the information and the results were just too good to ignore. It was probably because it all seemed so strange and unfamiliar. I am also sure that my path was supported by a group of people each giving of themselves, most often without my knowledge. To each I am thankful.

I would like to introduce you to our daughter-in-law, Erika. Her interest in healing modalities started in 1997, as I was struggling with my health. She, too, has struggled with her health, developing Fibromyalgia in her 20's. She has since studied Native American, Chinese and Ayurveda (India) healing approaches. It was she with our son, Al, who helped me with this information journey. It was she with our son, who developed the anti-inflammation herb combinations that have proven so valuable.

Erika and Al have developed, Green Heart, a full line of natural health products including salves, bath tea blends, massage oils, and topical aromatherapy blends. I have included some of her information on herbs and bath teas. Her informative full line product brochures are available with information on the benefits of essential oils, Qi Gong, herbal body wraps, salves, children and herbs, etc. (See Green Heart Natural Health Products in References.)

And watch for Erika's upcoming book.

Like Chris, I chose a very involved approach to regain my neurological health. At the time it was a quest for the best quality of life, but those actively involved choices have changed everything. They have been life changing choices. The Native Americans have a belief that the best medicine man is one who has been sick himself, that without this sickness, he would never truly understand and therefore would not be able to heal other people.

When in massage school, I was exposed to many wonderful people with many different alternative healing backgrounds. There were many cultures and viewpoints including herbs, massage, essential oils, nutrition diets, Qi Gong, energy work, social viewpoints and values, with Native American, Chinese and Ayurveda (India) healing approaches. But the biggest thing they did was to teach me to think... to teach me to explore... to teach me to try, and not to take "no cure" for an answer... and to be responsible for myself and my health.

It worked. Al and I started Green Heart Natural Health Products as an extension of this learning when people started asking us for the herbal products and the important information that was, and is, working for us.

The FDA does not always approve the use of herbs, essential oils, nutritional diets, mindsets/viewpoints, spirituality, meditation, and natural health. The human race has been successfully using all of these methods for thousands of years. It is only with the recent technical revolution that these long tested and used forms of healing have been abandoned. The following information is not meant to diagnose, treat, or cure. This is a cultural, humanitarian observation of how people have used alternative therapies for assisting the body to heal. You are responsible for your own health. Educate yourself, and open yourself to different viewpoints and cultures.

In using herbs, the name of a disease is not as important as the symptoms. The treatments for many discomforts and diseases overlap, and there may be many ways to get to the same result. It is even possible to see a disease forming before it affects life. Treat the little things before they become a big problem, thereby reducing the severity or preventing it entirely. We like to say "may you never know the disease you have prevented." Each person is unique. Their disease and healing journey will also be unique.

I feel the gentlest and safest way to start experimenting and exploring with herbs is in the bath. The dosages are very mild, yet very effective. They do not leave a heavy residue in the body so there are less chances of interferring with prescription drugs. And herbs are very affordable.

Also consider the viewpoint from traditional Chinese medicine. The body's ability to actually use what you eat, both herbs and nutritionally, depends on the functioning of the body's "energy" channels or meridians (Qi). It has come to my attention that there may be an underlying imbalance/damage in the meridians of the liver, stomach and heart/spirit in people with neurological problems that does not allow the body to use its food or herbs. With bath teas, we are going through the skin, bypassing the weakness, and drawing the vitamins, anti-oxidents and herbal values directly into the body.

Q. What is a Bath Tea?

A. A bath tea is any herb steeped in water that is then used to soak in or as a compress on the body.

Q. Do I drink Bath Teas?

A. Although not dangerous, bath teas were not blended for taste.

Q. How do I use a Bath Tea?

A. Put 1/4 cup, more or less, of the herbs in a cloth bag, nylon, sock, or tea ball. You can even use pre-made tea in bags, but this is more expensive. Fill the bath tub with about 3 inches of hot water. Add the herb bag and let it steep for 15 to 20 minutes. Just like a tea! Then finish filling the bath tub with the temperature water you would like and enjoy your soak.

Q. Why does a Bath Tea work?

A. The skin is the largest organ of the body. The skin is permeable which means that it can bring in nutrients, vitamins, and herbs (in liquid form) and expel toxins like uric and lactic acid, environmental pollutions and metabolic waste build-up out through the skin. The skin also brings in "bad" so be aware of skin products.

O. How quickly does a Bath Tea work?

A. You did not get sick overnight, this is something that has been building over time. Some people will see/feel changes in their body, or changes in behavior and stress tolerance in the first few weeks. Herbs help the body repair itself, it is never too early or too late to start using bath teas. People who benefit the most usually use bath teas 3 or 4 times a week.

Q. How do I choose the right herbs or Bath Tea Blends?

A. All herbs can be used as a bath tea. Some may be irritating to the skin in large quantities, like sage and cinnamon. Any herbs listed in the books as "tonics" are gentle and mild. "Medicinal" herbs have a stronger action than tonics. Medicinal herbs are more specialized and focused. By blending the two types you will achieve a more rounded support for the body. Each herb is a help for numerous body functions, and the body is a connected system. So when you improve the health in one area all parts will benefit. By listening to your body and researching, you will find your balance. You can start with our blends such as Sweet Dreams, Brain Support, Just for Kids, Joint Pain Anti-Inflammatory, Fibro-Aid, etc.

Q. Are there any cautions with Bath Teas?

A. All natural health products should be used with respect. Anything in excess can become an irritation to the body. As with all things you try, if an irritation should occur don't use! Some herbs (sage, cinnamon, and prickly ash bark) strongly increase circulation and heat in the body and can become a skin irritation.

Q. Can I use Bath Teas with very delicate people and children?

A. Yes, because you are not taking the herbs internally, they are very gentle. All the herbs listed as "tonic" are very mild and are a good place to start if you are uncertain. Nettle, lemon balm, red clover, lavender, plantain, catnip, dandelion and green tea are a few good choices.

Q. I don't have a bath, but have a medicinal need.

A. Bath teas can be used as a compress or a foot/hand soak. The bath will be the most effective because it covers more of your body. However, foot and leg soaks are very useful and important tools in health. Make the tea in a large mixing bowl or wash basin. Now you can soak just your hands or feet. For shoulders, neck, knees, elbows, or injury, dip a cloth into the tea and ring it out. Wrap over the problem area. Re-dip as necessary to keep warm.

Q. Can I add anything else to the Bath Tea?

A. Salts like Epsom or sea salt are added at the beginning and provide trace elements and minerals that the brain needs for nerve function and also to help with pain reduction. After the tea has steeped and the bath is ready, pure aloe vera gel or liquid can be added. Because you can also absorb the essential fatty acid's (the good Omega 3's) through your skin, 1/2 capful of flax oil (or one capsule), evening primrose or borage can be added. Baby oil and Vaseline are petroleum based and do not belong in good health care.

Q. What are some good herbs to use in the bath?

A. As you are in charge of your healing, I will give you some ideas on herbs to try. Enjoy referencing these and others. Note, be sure to rotate for a more complete coverage. Blend some of the gentle "tonic" herbs (see question 8) with these stronger "Medicinal" herbs: basil, damiana, ginger root, ginkgo, rosemary, gotu kola, St. John's wort, and skullcap, to name a few.

Healing energy

An important aspect of healing comes from feeling and using the universal spiritual healing energy around us. You can draw on this energy in many ways, and in you own way.

When a person is going through the turmoil of disease, it is often difficult to achieve this connection on your own. There are many modalities to help. Yoga, Qi Gong, Reiki, Prayer, Meditation, Bliss and Psyche are but a few. They all have one thing in common, which is to complement and complete the healing process. Some involve a more active participation, others require nothing more than "being."

We are in a great time in history. A time when many of the barriers among cultures are coming down. A time when we all can benefit from the knowledge each culture holds. We can once again gain what we lost in the seventeenth century, when the spiritual healing energy was separated from medicine. When the body was separated from the mind, soul, and emotions in healing.

As I stated in the beginning, our mother instilled in each of us the importance of knowledge and the natural instinct of caring for others. We, her children, each have developed this in our own way.

I am not the only one of my siblings to have to face Alzheimer's Disease. We each felt it with our mother. With the hereditary factor, we each have to come to terms with it.

Starting before I did, my younger brother, Ken, has sought to find a complementary art of healing. His journey has led him on a path along several avenues, culminating on Reiki.

In Reiki, Ken has found a technique for reducing stress and increasing relaxation which allows everyone to tap into an unlimited supply of "life force energy." In turn, improving health and enhancing the quality of life.

The knowledge of an unseen energy flowing through all living things connected directly to the quality of health has been part of the wisdom of many cultures since ancient times. Reiki is one way of increasing the energy with positive energy, thus clearing, straightening, and healing the energy pathways, allowing a more natural and healthy flow. Medical doctors are considering the role it plays in the functioning of the immune system and the healing process.

Reiki feels like a wonderful glowing radiance that flows through you and surrounds you. Reiki treats the whole person including body, emotions, mind, and spirit. Creating relaxation and feelings of peace, security, and well-being, it is a simple, natural and safe complement to healing that everyone can use. Reiki improves the results of medical and other therapy by reducing negative side effects, shortening healing time, reducing pain, reducing stress, and creating optimism. Reiki is both powerful and gentle.

Ken has chosen "caring for others" by teaching Reiki.

Ken Baum, Reiki Master Teacher
Appleton, WI   e-mail: energyki@aol.com

This has been my journey, seen through my eyes, remembered with my mind/body/soul. I am thankful for the support I have received allowing me to make this journey and back.

My husband, family and friends can tell you a different side to this journey. My husband alludes to happenings and events I have no memory of. Some doctors would say that with Alzheimer's Disease you do not know what is happening. And because I was "still in touch," I did not fit the norm. But you see, I was reporting what I knew, I could not report what I no longer remembered.

I realize now, only from what my family can tell me, that my short term memory was not functioning for quite some time. It was a lot worse than I knew, although I struggled every day to get back in control with the losses I could feel. They talk of my asking a question over and over. Of humoring me. Of telling me different answers so I'd go on a different path... for variety. I, of course, have no knowledge of this.

It is a very strange feeling to come back out of this separate life I was living. To hear from someone else what was actually happening... I know that there are years and events I will probably never get back. I rely on my feelings of something being "familiar" and trust my family.

My husband said today, he has lived with three different wives in one marriage. I am happy he stuck around to see this last one...

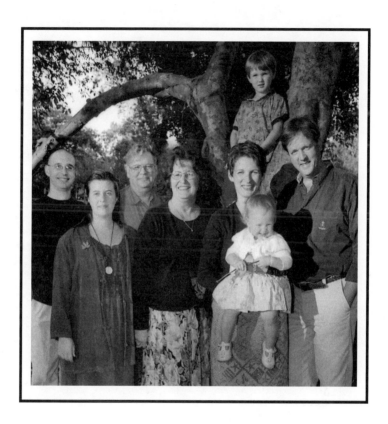

Al	Wade	Max in the tree,
with	with	Cassie with Ken
Erika	Chris	holding Maclean Rose

Our Growing Family
My Source of Love and Support
2004

Notes

Appendix

My bliss/energy place (from Chapter: II, page 34)

CHILDREN OF THE FARM

ENDLESS ADVENTURE - BEGINNING

It was an adventurous time
for young children born to the farm
Free to explore and
run with their imaginations.
Fifty years ago when all felt safer.

Born into the best of two worlds
as this farm was set at the edge of a city.
The "edge" was where the bus route was,
So as the children grew
the city awaited only a ride away.

An endless fantasy land
the farm held all the mysteries of
Life past with a promise of the future.

Its energies brought with those
Who had been there before –
waiting to be discovered and cherished…
Held and passed onto those that follow…

Children of the Farm

ENDLESS ADVENTURE - THE BARN

The rains come…
the barnyard becomes a muddy lake.
Follow the tractor tracks
walking, one bare foot in front of the other –
balance, don't miss.
Check for young heifers always ready to kick-up…
or the bull…
Always be ready to run Watchful child!

Surrounded by a cement moat –
like castles of kings and queens,
a navy of seed pods float across the cow tank.
Insect submarines dive to the green depths.
Watchful child feel the coldness of dungeons.
Off limits child –
too wonderful to resist!

Enter… the heavy wooden door,
stone walls, a ramp to take you deep.
The warm moist barn awaits.
Light filtering through windows aged with history.

Kittens hear the moment the door opens.
Older ones run forward
looking for a touch or treat –
newborn stay curled up under a board,
eyes barely open, Soft

Huge beasts plod through double doors
at the end of a cement runway.
Each knowing its resting place,
turning into its own stall.
Be alert! Watchful child.
Clanking of metal as stanchions
are closed about their heads.

Heads...
huge roving brown eyes
set in the middle of white.
Long tongues reaching out
for treasured ground grain
placed before them.

Hear the gurgle of water
released through mechanized dishes
awaiting on poles.

Swishing tails - child height...
move quickly Watchful child –
or be whipped in the face!

Giant, ancient beams, home to pigeons,
Crisscross the huge hall.
The upper barn holds hay and straw
of summers past.

Thick ropes twisted about beams,
hanging – inviting to a child to swing!
Trap doors hidden beneath floor boards
open to the life of the barn below.
Watchful child - beware.

Climb to the top of the golden straw-
a coat of dust settled on top.
Sink knee deep in silken threads –
A child's delight!

Carefully walk on boards let loose
To the room of bins.
Danger is everywhere – Watchful child
As the suffocating grain
encloses anyone who steps into it.

Reach and climb wooden steps
Not touching the floor.
Explore the old –
find the past in the room left in peace.
Old metal and leather shapes
of a useful life gone by.
Child - you have found
the forgotten life of the horses,
Long gone.

A tower to the castle,
Climb it high!
Stretch your legs and arms – Reach –
Do not look down Watchful child.

Wooden boards face your eyes –
cement and stone surround you child
as you climb higher…
Crawl through into the safe circular hall -
Echo the voices of young.

Flapping of wings like beating rugs,
Cooing multi-shades of brown and white,
The doves scare off. Ground feed at your feet…
You are in the silo of old.
A wonder.

Stretch those small arms and legs…
Reach… Reach…
Face laying in the feed…
Feet and legs dangling over the edge
Into the vertical tower
that was so easy to climb up.
Reach…Watchful child
Find each rung, climb down
All the way to the bottom!

Crawl out through the window
at the base – walk around to the back,
Sit upon the narrow ledge,
Feet dangling – fresh air blowing in your face.
Tell secrets.
See the fields in the distance, barnyard below
Weeds growing up to reach your toes.
Rest…

The hill, Our hill – A mountain to little feet.
A run to the bottom.
The hill making little legs run faster… faster…
and faster… Out of breath!

Or find the sharp side, crawl up it
Aided by little child's hands gripping grass.
A wooden post to help the way.

Watchful child – snow covered
It becomes the Alps…
Slide - on runners of metal
steering out a curve.

Or ride the wild bronco –
An uncontrolled run made with the curve
of a barrel slat, a seat nailed in place.

When the crisp winter adds a coat of ice –
all children tumble onto a long toboggan
and ride to the bottom!
Our mountain –
Our exploration!

This is the Barn of a Watchful Child…
Pulsed with life and death,
Old and new,
Change and unchange.

ENDLESS ADVENTURE - THE FIELDS

Edged by fences
Rutted by tractor tires and hooves
Finely tuned by bicycle tires
spun and swirled. The lane
Connecting fields and running on for forever.

Pack a bag of crackers and jam
Watchful child, and take a trip.
Parts are dry sand with a rocky edge
others soft with moss in the shade of a tree.

A lonely aged tree
stands at the mid point.
Each piece of rough and shaped bark
a story of the past.
Its ill formed branches
the legend of drought and flood.
Each year bearing its fruit
A treasure to little hands
Who else stopped beneath this tree Watchful child?

Continue on, the lane becomes
A roller coaster of uneven land.
Out of breath!

Reach two small shaped crab apple trees.
Tiny red tart fruit at its feet.
Sentries at the far end of the lane.
Buzzing with life
as bees nest in its womb.
Little relief from the sun.
Not visited often.

The lane comes alive
With the thunder of hooves,
Parched tongues hanging
Ready to be relieved of their heavy loads.
Run Watchful child, heart racing
Duck under the fence, escape!
The beasts of the barn return from the fields.

Enter the flowing field of oats
Walk through it.
When it is knee high in June
the last day of school
Come home early from the school picnic
To tenderly remove the choking
Yellow mustard from its roots.
Green now – Golden by the end of summer
To become a silken nest of straw
In the upper barn when harvested in fall.

Find the endless pastures.
Enter the "plains" where
Indians could come passing by
or buffalo – perhaps elephants led by Tarzan.

Dry cow pies hold the makings
for a fishing trip with worms galore,
Fresh cow pies like evil quick sand.

The land rolls on carved with
Paths worn firm
Cows always in single file
heading back to the barn.
Paths that kick up dust in summer heat
and run of mud after a rainfall.

Protected by barbed wire
Pulsing with electrical current
the field of corn.
Be careful Watchful child
or you will loose your way.

Corn growing to the sky
taking with it north and south,
east and west.
Sharp edges of green scrape,
Cutting face and bare arms
Yet feel fuzzy.
Appearing friendly with a dusting of fine blossoms,
But always standing firm and overbearing.

Among the tall grasses at a field's edge
Lay the last of a great tree.
Cut with a mighty hand,
Stump and log head high.

Come Watchful child
and play upon me.
What will you be today?
A doctor nursing his patients
with tools plucked from my shredded stump?
A sailor with his ship's mates playing "I spy"?
Perhaps a cook or a pilot.

These are the Fields of a Watchful Child...
Endless to little feet
Waiting to release their hidden treasures.

ENDLESS ADVENTURE - THE ORCHARD
White and pink blossoms
One over lapping the other.
Tall grasses at Watchful child's feet.
An orchard of fruit trees, treasured.

Explore the mushrooms so huge
Little arms cannot wrap around them,
Sitting like white balls…
Waiting and waiting –
For what?

Beehives stacked to heights –
sentinels among the growing.
Busy with life, left to themselves.
Danger, Watchful child

Next, a "Honey House" now standing quiet,
The factory for the bees energies.
Open the door carefully, stuck half way
Always dark, enter with a flashlight.

To the left a metal platform and tank
Once collected the honey.
Shine to the right, only storage for old items.
Explore Watchful child,
Feel the presence of those before you.

Through the orchard a small red building
Brought to life each spring
with the delivery of boxes alive with energy.
Peeping boxes delivered in the mail
with little holes in them.

Run to the small building Watchful child
Clean and warm it… Shoo away the varmints.
Its life has arrived!

Huddle close – watch them run child
Little, yellow mounds of fluff.
Pick out the males –
Their fancy skin red top.

Watchful child, care for them
Warm them under the ring of light
Nurse them…
Watch the feathers grow turning to white.

One day, open the little doors
with the ramps leading outside.
Watch as they catch bugs off the ground
made soft with years of chicks before them.
Fenced in so as not to run away.

A craggy tree becomes their perch by summer's end.
Find the eggs hidden in wild nests.
By fall they are caught
and brought to the big hen house.

The BIG hen house
Where matrons rule.
Two doors swing on hinges to enter.
Step up as the years raise the floor level.
Boxes all on end holding nests, Careful
Watchful child - these matrons rule.

"Keep quiet!" is uttered by Grandmother
least you scare them.
Glass and wooden eggs
lay in prepared nests
encouraging young hens.

Chickens perch on wooden rails
running the length of the room.
Light seeps through old windows,
screened outside with overgrown flowers.
Not a place to stay Watchful child.

Attached is a building
Which long ago held laughing children
studying their ABC's
Then torn down board by board
and rebuilt on this farm
To hold the tools of farming.

The glorious school bell re-hung
on the floor above.
Climb those steps, Watchful child,
Not quite rebuilt in proper order
large and small
spaced close and far.
Explore the equipment of years past.
Make room - hang a hoop
Now it's a basketball court!

This is the orchard of a Watchful child....
Ever busy with adult accomplishments
And children's imagination.

ENDLESS ADVENTURE - THE GARDENS

Run your feet, child, through
Warm black dirt, newly tilled
Like sand on a beach
The fine dirt awaits its life.

Dig small holes dropping 4 seeds
Cover, dig, plant, cover, dig,
Plant, over and over.
Get down on your knees, child
Carefully shape the row, sprinkle
fine seed hardly felt in tiny hands.
Gently, gently cover and pat tenderly.

Child, follow behind the shovel
Watch it dig and lift – drop in the cut potato
before the shovel leaves the ground
Follow - Follow - Follow.

Brother plant the peanuts
Will they grow? Will they taste good?

Watch the rain soak the earth bringing life.
A good drenching rain is
needed for the last planting.
Leave your shoes in the house, Watchful child.
Roll up your pant legs. Gather
the round dowels and we will begin.

Punch a hole in the muddy earth
Take a seedling giving it a new home.
Mud squeezing between your toes
Mud giving life to a new plant
growing tall and green, or round and fat.

Share a row of luscious berries
with your mother, child.
Small arms stretching
to reach as far as mother's do.
Talk of special thoughts held dear.
Pans from the kitchen filled with red
Sweetness, as child and mother stoop along the rows.
Spring rains have done well in their nurturing.
Brother, put up a table by the road.
Sell the strawberries.

Tie small pails around your waist, child.
Set little wicker baskets in place
stained from years past. Fill with raspberries
snatched from canes of green.
Watch for little black bugs
buried deep in a hollow center.

Tie your hair up tight and sit
with Grandmother beneath
a bush hanging with clumps of ripe fruit.
Strip the fruit into huge metal bowls held in laps.
Small round currents cleaned and added to jams.

Vines twisted around wooden guides
stand parallel to the lane only a fence
and burdock leaves between.
Giving of its fruit in the fall,
grapes canned or made into jelly

Watchful child, climb high into the tree!
Reach for its bounty before the winds
shake it loose to fall and bruise.
Buckets tied to a rope, lowered and
emptied below to be pulled back up
Filled again and again
Pies, sauce, and cakes await the apples each year.

Gladiolas, zinnias, daisies
The flowers of a farming wife. Roses on
Trellis sentries at the front door,
Petunias edging the walks
All dress up a working farm.

These are the Gardens of a Watchful Child
Bringing nourishment and comfort
To those that live there.

References and Information

An excellent source for quality herbs, lotions, salves, herbal bath teas, aromatherapy, books, massage and Qi Gong.

Green Heart Natural Health Products
PO Box 571
Appleton, WI 54912
(920) 882-1277
www.greenheartnaturalhealth.com
(See order blank in back of book)
> Distributed by: Galaxy Science & Hobby Center, Inc
> 1607 N. Richmond St, Appleton, WI 54911
> (920) 730-9220

Reiki Energy Work

Ken Baum, Reiki Master Teacher
Appleton, WI
www.energyki@aol.com

Quality of Life Therapies

Morris Friedell
http://members.aol.com/MorrisFF/vision.html
http://members.aol.com/MorrisFF/index.html

Self-Publishing Services
Raven Tree Press, LLC
Dawn Jeffers and Amy Crane Johnson
200 S. Washington St. Suite 306
Green Bay, WI 54301
920-438-1605   www.raventreepress.com

Information on Herbs & Health

Your local Herb, Holistic, or Nutrition Centers.

The Green Pharmacy, James A Duke, Ph.D. Rodale Press,
   Pennsylvania. 1997

Planetary Herbology, Dr. Michael Tierra, C.A., N.D., O.M.D.
   Lotus Press, Twin Lakes, WI

Prescription for Nutritional Healing, James Balch, M.D. and
   Phyllis A. Balch, C.N.C. Avery Publishing, N.Y. 1997

Taber's Cyclopedic Medical Dictionary, Edition 17. F.A. Davis
   Company, PA

Ultimate Herb and Nutritional Reference, Karen Waggoner
   Royal Oaks Publishing, Mo. 2001

The Herb Quarterly, (A publication). 1041 Shary Circle,
   Concord, CA 94518 www,herbquarterly.com

Alternative Medicine Foundation (A Web Site). Sponsored by
   a Maryland nonprofit group.
   www.amfoundation.org

National Center for Complementary and Alternative Medicine.
   A division of The National Institute of Health.
   www.nccam.nih.gov

U.S. National Library of Medicine and The National Institute
   of Health.
   medlineplus.gov

Alzheimer Disease International
   www.alz.co.uk

Clinical Trials
   http://clinicaltrials.gov

Books

Blaylock, Russell, M.D. *Excitotoxins The Taste That Kills*.
    New Mexico: Health Press, 1997.
    PO Box 37470, Albuquerque, 87176

Chopra, Deepak, M.D. *Quantum Healing, Exploring the
    Frontiers of Mind/Body Medicine*. New York: Bantam
    Books, 1990.

Khalsa, Dharma Singh, M.D., with Stauth, Cameron. *Brain
    Longevity*. New York: Warner Books, Inc. 1997

Newmark, Thomas and Schulick, Paul. *Beyond Aspirin*.
    Arizona: Hohm Press, 2000.
    PO Box 2501, Prescott, 86302, 800-381-2700)

Norden, Michael, M.D. *Beyond Prozac*. New York: Harper
    Collins, 1996

Orloff, Judith, M.D. *Second Sight*. New York: Warner Books,
    Inc., 1996

Pert, Candace, Ph.D. *Molecules of Emotion*. New York:
    Simon and Schuster, Inc. 1999

Pollen, Daniel A. *Hannah's Heirs, The Quest for the Genetic
    Origins of Alzheimer's Disease*. New York: Oxford
    University Press, Inc., 1996

Redfield, James. *The Celestine Prophecy*. New York:
    Warner Books, 1993

Stein, Donald with Brailowsky, Simon and Will, Bruno.
    Brain Repair. New York: Oxford University Press, Inc.,
    1995.

Eades, Michael R. M.D. and Eades, Mary Dan, M.D.
    Protein Power. New York: Bantam Books, 1998

To Find Researchers in your Area,
Contact the National Alzheimer's Association

National Alzheimer's Association
919 N. Michigan Avenue, #1000
Chicago, IL 60611-1676
(800) 272-3900
www.alz.org

Dr. Benjamin R. Brooks, Professor
Department of Neurology
University of Wisconsin Hospital and Clinics
600 Highland Ave.
Madison, WI 53792

Dr. Janelle L. Copper
The Memory Center
Affinity Health System
2700 W. 9th Ave, Suite 203
Oshkosh, WI 54902
Dietary Lipids in the Aetiology of Alzheimer's Disease,
Implications for Therapy 2003

Dr. Bird
Alzheimer's Disease Research Center
University of Washington
Genetics Section
VA Medical Center
GRECC 182B
1660 S. Columbian Way
Seattle, WA 98108-1597
(800) 745-4511

Wisconsin Alzheimer's Institute
University of WI - Madison
7818 Big Sky Drive, Suite 215
Madison, WI 53719
608-829-3300 Fax: 608-829-3315
E-mail:waimail@wai.wisc.edu Web: www.medsch.wisc.edu/wai

Index

H

Hannah's Heirs, 132-137, 157
Heal, 27-28, 50, 66-72, 77, 88, 162
Heart disease, 121, 154, 157, 203, 231
Heart's Code, The, 162
Herbal tea bath, 198-199, 202, 292-297
Herbs, 160, 265
Highly Sensitive Person, The, 98, 159
Hippocampus, 88
Holy Basil, 190-198
Hops, 193
Hope, 30, 156, 160, 265, 286-287
Hostage Brain, 156
How, The, 41
Hum, 29-30, 264-265, 271
Huntington's disease, 205-229, 231
Hydrolyzed protein, 205-229
Hyperinsulinemia, 154
Hyperlipidemia, 157
Hypothalamus, 208-229

I

Inflammation, 154, 181, 186-192, 203, 270-271
Inflammatory, 100
Instincts, 155
Intelligence, 28, 70, 162
Intuition, 66, 71, 75, 161

J

Jonathan Livingston Seagull, 31

L

L-cysteine, 204-230, 271
Laughter, 157, 198
Lavender, 198
Lecithin, 278
Lemon grass, 198
Life's Extension, 125
LOAD study, 253
Love Is..., 141

M

Magnesium, 205-229
Map, 138
Masters of Wit, 57
Medical diary, 281
Meditation, 28-29, 68, 72, 89, 91, 265
Melatonin, 100, 191-198
Memory, 45, 86, 88, 103, 121, 127, 131, 158, 160, 191
Metabolism, 48, 213-229
   cellular, 88
Mild cognitive impairment, 86, 91
Mitochondria, 213-229, 279
Molecules of Emotion, 157
Molybdenum, 182
Motor/muscle testing, 93-94, 266, 280
MS, 231
MSG (monosodium glutamate), 204-230, 271, 279
My Child, The Farm Responds, 256

Green Heart Natural Health Products

We have put together two sample packets of anti-inflammatory and emotional support products.

Small Sample Packet: $12.00

1 oz Auntie's Anti #1 Topical Anti-inflammatory
1 oz Auntie's Anti #2 Topical Anti-inflammatory
> Essential oils in a ready to use topical aloe and jojoba base. Originally designed for neurological support, but also works great for pain and inflammation of all types. Use as a body splash for fragrance, blend with lotions to scent them, or use where medicinally needed. (Anti-inflammatory, antioxidant, respiratory and emotional support, circulation, pain, memory.)

2 oz Bath Tea "Brain Builders"
2 oz Bath Tea "Joint Pain PM" Anti-inflammatory
2   Tea Bags
Free 1/4 oz First Aide Herbal Salve
> Natural oils, bees wax, herbs and essential oils.

Large Sample Packet $40.00

2 oz Auntie's Anti #1 Topical Anti-inflammatory
2 oz Auntie's Anti #2 Topical Anti-inflammatory
2 oz Bath Tea "Brain Builder"
2 oz Bath Tea "Joint Pain PM" Anti-inflammatory
2 oz Bath Tea "Stressed Out" Nerve protector
2 oz Bath Tea "Sniffles"
2   Tea Bags
2 oz Lavender Water Essential Oil Room & Body Spray
> Essential oils diluted in distilled water. Supports emotional & mental health, soothing, relaxation aide.

1   Organic, Cold Pressed, Flax 1000 mg "Health from the Sun" soft gels. 100 count. Add to the bath tea soak or as a supplement.
1   Lotion sample. Use as is or blend with Auntie's Anti for full body coverage.
Free 1/4 oz First Aide and 1/8 oz Summer Solstice Salves

Green Heart Natural Health Products
PO Box 571, Appleton, WI 54912 (920) 882-1277
www.greenheartnaturalhealth.com

REPLY CARD - Please send the following:

____ *Alzheimer's Averted: A Path to Survival* $25.00

Green Heart Natural Health Products:
____   Small Sample Packet: $12.00   (see page 326)
____   Large Sample Packet $40.00   (see page 326)
____   Free Green Heart mini catalog of products.

____ Information on seminars/speaking engagements

____ Please add my name to the mailing list for
future books by Elemental Basic Publishing.

Shipping: U.S. $4.00 for first book/product, and $2.00 for each additional book/product. International: $9.00 for first book/product, and $5.00 for each additional book/product.

Sales Tax: (Wisconsin) Please add appropriate Wisconsin tax.

Name:_____

Address:_____

City, State, Zip:_____

Telephone_____

Payment total $_____   Check____ Money Order_____

Please charge my Visa____   MC____ Discover____ AmExp___

Card Number_____ Exp Date_____

Signature_____

ELEMENTAL BASIC PUBLISHING
P.O. Box 571
Appleton, WI 54912
www.elementalbasicpub.com   (920) 882-1277
Please allow 3 weeks for delivery. Thank you

Also available at: Galaxy Science & Hobby Center, Inc
1607 N. Richmond St., Appleton, WI 54911, (920) 730-9220

REPLY CARD - Please send the following:

____ *Alzheimer's Averted: A Path to Survival* $25.00

Green Heart Natural Health Products:
____   Small Sample Packet: $12.00   (see page 326)
____   Large Sample Packet $40.00   (see page 326)
____   Free Green Heart mini catalog of products.

____ Information on seminars/speaking engagements

____ Please add my name to the mailing list for
         future books by Elemental Basic Publishing.

Shipping: U.S. $4.00 for first book/product, and $2.00 for each additional book/product. International: $9.00 for first book/product, and $5.00 for each additional book/product.

Sales Tax: (Wisconsin) Please add appropriate Wisconsin tax.

Name:_____

Address:_____

City, State, Zip:_____

Telephone_____ E-mail_____

Payment total $_____   Check____ Money Order_____

Please charge my Visa____ MC____ Discover____ AmExp___

Card Number_____ Exp Date_____

Signature_____

ELEMENTAL BASIC PUBLISHING
P.O. Box 571
Appleton, WI 54912
www.elementalbasicpub.com   (920) 882-1277
Please allow 3 weeks for delivery.   Thank you

Also available at: Galaxy Science & Hobby Center, Inc
1607 N. Richmond St., Appleton, WI 54911, (920) 730-9220